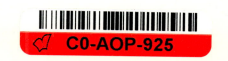

Family Therapy
Education and Supervision

THE *JOURNAL OF PSYCHOTHERAPY & THE FAMILY* SERIES:

Family Therapy Education and Supervision

Fred P. Piercy
Editor

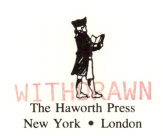

The Haworth Press
New York • London

Family Therapy Education and Supervision has also been published as *Journal of Psychotherapy & the Family,* Volume 1, Number 4, Winter 1985/86.

The Haworth Press, Inc., 28 East 22 Street, New York, NY 10010-6194
EUROSPAN/Haworth, 3 Henrietta Street, London WC2E 8LU England

Library of Congress Cataloging-in-Publication Data
Main entry under title:

Family therapy education and supervision.

    Also published as: Journal of psychotherapy & the family, v. 1, no. 4, winter 1985/86.
    Bibliography: p.
    1. Family psychotherapy—Study and teaching—Addresses, essays, lectures. 2. Family therapists—Supervision of—Addresses, essays, lectures.
I. Piercy, Fred P. [DNLM: 1. Family Therapy—education.
W1 J0859C v.1 no. 4 / WM 18 F198]
RC488.5.F339 1986   616.89'156'071 85-21958
ISBN 0-86656-510-8
ISBN 0-86656-511-6 (pbk.)

Family Therapy Education and Supervision

Journal of Psychotherapy & the Family
Volume 1, Number 4

CONTENTS

EDITORIAL NOTE

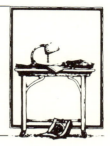

This collection, entitled FAMILY THERAPY EDUCATION AND SUPERVISION, is the fourth issue in the *Journal of Psychotherapy & the Family's* inaugural year of publication. Its thrust is quite consistent with the Journal's aim, which is to provide the most well written, accurate, authoritative, and relevant information on the practice of psychotherapy with families.

Most observers would agree that professional clinical intervention with families has enjoyed steady growth for the last two decades. And within the last several years family-centered services have evolved from a few university centers and treatment programs to their current widespread popularity. More than ever, professionals are being *trained* to work with families. The disciplines that train psychotherapists increasingly are embracing the family as a unit of analysis and intervention, and implementing procedures and standards for family assessment and treatment. For example, social workers, who have traditionally viewed the family as a primary unit of intervention, have just recently begun using systemic concepts and interventions. Not until 1984 did the American Psychological Association establish a section on "Family Psychology". Similarly, in the last few years the American Association of Counseling and Development formed a family therapy interest committee within its Association of Counselor Education and Supervision.

Yet, very little has been published which provides guidelines for *training* these new family clinicians—either through graduate programs, institutes, or other continuing education. And this is precisely why the collection of papers to follow is so vital to psychotherapy. In this collection, edited by Dr. Fred P. Piercy, are papers from some of the leading educators and supervisors from psychology, psychiatry, education, and family therapy focusing on such central issues of family therapy training, as supervision, theory building, choosing family therapy training, training in

family therapy as a profession versus a specialty, feminist views of training, post-graduate training, and others. As specialization grows within
the established fields of psychotherapy and as the new psychotherapy
field of family therapy emerges, this collection should become an important resource.

Dr. Piercy is quickly becoming a leader in the area of family therapy
training, through both his writings and his work as an educator and supervisor. He has written numerous papers on such topics as graduate family
therapy education and supervision, assessment, ethics, and family therapy practice and research. Moreover, he has won several teaching awards,
and many of his students have published in the leading journals and have
won nationally competitive research awards. He has been a member of
the Advisory Committee to the Commission on Accreditation for Family
Therapy Education, and has been an accreditation site visitor to numerous
universities. Dr. Piercy also has held many leadership positions within
the American Association for Marriage and Family Therapy at both the
state and national level. In addition to being on the Editorial Council of
the *Journal of Psychotherapy & the Family,* Dr. Piercy is also on the
editorial board of the *Journal of Marital and Family Therapy* and the
Journal of Strategic and Systemic Therapies.

This edited collection is a compliment to Dr. Piercy's impressive cre-
dentials in this field. No other collection has included so many key individuals knowledgable about family therapy training. For example, Robert
Beavers is the incoming president of the American Association for Marriage and Family Therapy and the former chair of the AAMFT Commission on Supervision, Florence Kaslow is a former editor of the *Journal of
Marital and Family Therapy.* Bunny Duhl, Howard Liddle, Beavers, and
Kaslow all direct nationally prominent family therapy institutes, and Al
Hovestadt, Jim Keller, Doug Sprenkle, and Liddle have all been directors
of family therapy doctoral programs. Moreover, all of these people are
regarded as authorities in family therapy training.

In addition, some of the less known authors in this volume make new
and significant contributions to the training literature. Dorothy Wheeler,
Judy Avis, Lori Miller, and Sita Chaney, for example, look at family
therapy training through feminist eyes, and provide many useful suggestions to trainers. Similarly, Phil Sutton's "insider" view of both a family
therapy doctoral program and a post graduate training center raise many
important training issues.

In sum, this volume is a rare "one of a kind" that is at the same time
provocative, informative, current, and perhaps most importantly, useful
to the practitioner/trainer.

Charles R. Figley, Ph.D
Editor

Family Therapy
Education and Supervision

Preface

The explosion called family therapy has had a profound impact on mental health treatment. And the dust has not settled yet. Family therapy books and journals are multiplying exponentially, as is membership in organizations like the American Association for Marriage and Family Therapy (AAMFT) and the American Family Therapy Association. With all the current interest in family therapy, it is not surprising that graduate and post graduate family therapy training programs are proliferating, and family therapy courses are beginnning to be offered in departments of psychology, psychiatry, social work, psychiatric nursing, professional counseling, and clinical pastoral education.

Professional training programs accredited by AAMFT support and underline the emerging status of family therapy as a distinct mental health profession. At the same time, since a large part of every psychotherapist's caseload involves marriage and family related presenting problems, other types of training in family therapy are becoming important. The present volume on family therapy education and supervision is prepared with both the psychotherapist and family therapist in mind. The subjects are written from objective, subjective, theoretical, practical and political vantage points and span such topics as graduate and post graduate education and supervision, family therapy theory building, feminism and family therapy training, and future directions of family therapy education. Many provide a first-hand view of training approaches that the reader may use as a trainer or participant. In all, the papers reflect well the vitality, breadth, depth, excitement and creativity that are evident in today's family therapy education and supervision.

In the first paper, Fred Piercy and Doug Sprenkle discuss their integrative approach to teaching graduate level family therapy theory in a university setting. These authors make a strong case for teaching major theoretical models in ways that invite both thoughtful criticism and potential integration. Family therapy educators should find their illustrative training procedures useful. Moreover, single-theory trainers should be challenged to consider the advantages of a more integrative training approach.

Robert Beavers, in the next paper, presents an overview of family therapy supervision that also serves as a "consumer's guide" to therapists wishing to receive family therapy supervision. While Beavers' characterizations are painted in broad strokes, family therapists, no doubt, will recognize many of the likenesses that emerge.

1

David Fenell and Alan Hovestadt grapple with several important practical and political questions. Is family therapy a profession or a professional specialty? And what implications does this issue have for family therapy training in academic settings? Fenell and Hovestadt, while personally supporting the view of family therapy as a profession, suggest a three-level model relevant to graduate academic programs viewing family therapy as either a profession, professional specialty, or area for elective study.

Phillip Sutton offers the reader an "insider's" view of family therapy training. While his experiences at Purdue and the Philadelphia Child Guidance Clinic may not generalize to all settings, his comparison of these two experiences raises important training issues for anyone seeking an appropriate family therapy training experience.

Papers five through eight are on specific training procedures. The first of these breaks new ground in a virtually ignored, yet important area of family therapy training—that of supervision from a feminist perspective. Dorothy Wheeler, Judith Meyers Avis, Lorie Miller, and Sita Chaney provide a compelling rationale for feminist-informed family therapy supervision, and identify conceptual, perceptual, and executive skills related to feminist issues in family therapy.

In the next paper, Kaslow describes in detail a six-day post-graduate institute model for training family therapy professionals. While Kaslow relates distinct advantages of an intensive format at an idyllic location, many of her training activities also may be applied to more traditional family therapy training settings.

Next, James Keller and Howard Protinsky present a unique approach to family therapy supervision. In their integrative model, they use the process of the supervision group to help supervisees become aware of and deal with family of origin patterns that may inhibit their therapeutic effectiveness. Their fresh approach to applying Bowenian concepts in the on-going process of group supervision is compelling, and should challenge blind allegiance to live supervision as the *only* useful family therapy supervision format.

Bunny Duhl describes an intriguing integrative approach to training in systems thinking developed at the Boston Family Institute (BFI). She discusses BFI's experiential/cognitive blend of training in terms of Piagetian theory, learning styles, and exercises meant to stimulate "right and left brain" functioning. Her model connects trainees' personal experiences with systems theory and therapeutic skills. While techniques are emphasized in many other approaches to supervision and training, Duhl reminds us that people are, in the final analysis, the instruments of change and that the training of whole persons/therapists is a challenging and exciting enterprise.

In the final paper, Howard Liddle challenges us to broaden our view of family therapy training. Liddle contends that, as family therapy trainers, we should define our roles with a sensitivity to the multiple contexts within which we work and live. His provocative questions on our roles in both family therapy and non-family therapy contexts should stimulate us to consider the far reaching influence we might have in the education and application of systems ideas.

The "department" sections of this collection are meant to serve as resources for readers interested in supervision and training information. First is a list of family therapy training programs accredited by the Commission on Accreditation for Marriage and Family Therapy Education. Next are book and videotape reviews by Mark Hirschmann, Roger Laird, Nick Aradi, and Karen Hernandez. And finally, Marcia Brown, Mark Hirschmann, John Lasley, and Cricket Steinweg have compiled an excellent annotated bibliography of key articles on the supervision and training of family therapists.

Fred P. Piercy, Ph.D.
Guest Editor

Family Therapy Theory Building:
An Integrative Training Approach

Fred P. Piercy
Douglas H. Sprenkle

ABSTRACT. Our approach to graduate family therapy education involves the teaching of the major theoretical models in a way that invites
both thoughtful criticism and potential integration into one's own personal
theory of family therapy. The purpose of this paper is to briefly decribe the
rationale for our integrative training procedures, and to present several illustrative examples of learning activities designed to stimulate theoretical
criticism and creative integration.

Family therapy education and supervision have a short history. Just
three decades ago, family therapy, then a revolutionary process, began
with the work of creative pioneers such as Nathan Ackerman, Carl
Whitaker, John Eldenkin Bell, Murray Bowen, and others. A network of
iconoclastic family therapists developed, each proposing somewhat different theoretical formulations and intervention techniques. Training initially resembled an apprenticeship, with promising neophytes observing,
working with, and generally sitting at the feet of the masters (Kaslow,
1977; Nichols, 1979). Even today, family therapy "superstars" (Pittman, 1983) demonstrate their skills to large audiences and often are
wisked in and out of workshops like contemporary rock stars.

To be sure, family therapy education also has taken on a more formalized air, owing largely to the advent of family therapy training centers
and graduate programs. Requisite skills are beginning to be specified
(Allred & Kersey, 1977; Cleghorn & Levin, 1973; Falicov, Constantine
& Breunlin, 1981; Garrigan & Bambrick, 1977; Piercy, Laird &
Mohammed, 1983; Tomm & Wright, 1979) and procedures have begun
to be operationalized for the teaching of family therapy skills and concepts (Constantine, Fish & Piercy, 1984; Liddle, 1980; Liddle & Saba,
1982; Liddle & Schwartz, 1983; Piercy & Sprenkle, 1984). Moreover,

---

Fred P. Piercy, Ph.D., is an Associate Professor of Family Therapy and Director of Training
and Research, Family Therapy Doctoral Program, Department of Child Development and Family
Studies, Purdue University, West Lafayette, IN 47907.

Douglas H. Sprenkle, Ph.D., is an Associate Professor of Family Therapy and the Director of
the Family Therapy Doctoral Program at the same institution.

nontherapy courses have been suggested as important components in the
well rounded education of family therapists (Piercy & Sprenkle, 1983;
Sprenkle & Piercy, 1984). Research on family therapy training procedures has been proposed (Kniskern & Gurman, 1979; Liddle, 1982; Liddle
& Halpin, 1978) but relatively few studies on family therapy training
have been conducted to date (e.g. Mohammed & Piercy, 1983; Winkle,
Piercy & Hovestadt, 1981).

How one should best teach family therapy will continue to be debated
and hopefully researched. Important questions related to family therapy
education include: What school or schools of family therapy should be
taught? Should one family therapy model be taught in isolation, or are
there advantages to teaching several models? Should theoretical integration be encouraged or discouraged?

Many family therapy trainers teach one model that is clear, theoretically consistent, and relatively easy to master (Bowen, 1978; Liddle, 1980,
1982; Liddle & Saba, 1982). Purist trainers emphasize certain risks inherent in mixing theoretical models. These risks include the incompata-
bility of various theoretical tenets, the difficulty of teaching an integrated
model, the utopian expectation ("all things for all people") that such a
model generates, and the lack of rigor and consistency that an integrated
model might spawn (Fraser, 1982; Liddle, 1982). Also, when training
programs are short, it is considered more simple and practical to teach
one existing model well.

We believe that these are all legitimate risks worthy of attention. Yet
we are concerned with the potential wealth of useful information denied
students when only one model is taught. Also, not enough is known about
the relative efficacy of the predominant models of family therapy to judge
one to be clearly superior to another. In our own approach to training we
attempt to teach each of the major family therapy theories in a way that invites both thoughtful criticism and potential integration of selected assumptions into the students' evolving personal theory of family therapy.
The purpose of this paper is to briefly describe the rationale for our integrative training procedures, and to present several examples of learning
activities designed to stimulate theoretical criticism and creative integration.

RATIONALE FOR INTEGRATIVE THERAPY AND TRAINING

We affirm the advantages of an integrative family therapy model identified by Lebow (1984). Lebow states that integrative approaches a) draw
from a broader theoretical base than do purist models, b) allow for
greater flexibility in the treatment of any given individual or family, c)

are more applicable to a broader client population then more narrowly focused approaches, d) allow for a better fit between therapist and treatment approach, e) make it possible to combine the major benefits of specific approaches, f) bring greater objectivity into the selection of change strategies, since there is less investment in one particular model, and g) can be readily adapted to include new techniques.

We also affirm the importance of an integrative *training* approach to doctoral level family therapy education. While learning one family therapy model exclusively is often appropriate in post graduate workshops or training institutes after trainees have already been exposed to a variety of models, we believe that a doctoral program in family therapy should be committed to a broad exposure to the field. Therefore, in our four-course theory sequence we enthusiastically teach the major approaches to family therapy, but in an atmosphere where criticism, skepticism, and creative inquiry also are encouraged. Moreover, all students take a general course in theory construction in which they learn the characteristics of a good theory as well as the skills of theory criticism and construction. In essence, we want to *expose* discerning students to the field rather than *impose* any one model. In our theory sequence, theoretical underpinnings, interventions, and research data are examined for strategic, structural, behavioral, transgenerational, communicational, and experiential family therapies.

Structured learning activities are used in each of our theory courses to encourage the contrasting of theoretical assumptions, not only between theories, but also between the student's own theoretical assumptions and those posited by particular family therapy schools. In these learning activities, we attempt to personally involve the student by stretching his/her own assumptions of the world and by encouraging the student to test assumptions of a particular model against his/her own world view and lived experience. We are, as Duhl (1983) suggests, attempting to teach both from the "inside out" and from the "outside in". We believe that the resultant process is one of informed personal theory building, based on exposure to the prominent theorists, practitioners, and researchers in the field.

In essence, we are attempting to combine content-centered and person-centered teaching approach to educate discerning scholars to avoid the pitfalls of being either a true believer or a wide-eyed eclectic (Piercy, 1984). We challenge students to be theoretically consistent, but accept the legitimacy of applying intervention strategies from a variety of models to meet theory-specified therapy goals.

Further, students are encouraged to see their emerging theoretical tenets not as "truth" but as mid-level constructs which help translate a systemic paradigm into clinical practice (Sluzki, 1983). As such, we hope that students will avoid the hubris that has characterized much family therapy theory. In emphasizing that the map is not the territory, each student is encouraged to see his/her theory as a helpful (albeit incomplete) guide that reflects a portion of reality and logically leads to certain intervention strategies. Like any theory, it is not tested against "truth," but is evaluated on the extent that it is heuristic, parsimonious, consistent, and above all, useful.

Since the student who is developing his/her own theory is necessarily an explorer and pioneer him/herself, the integrative family therapies of others (e.g., Duhl & Duhl, 1981; Stanton 1981; Pinsof, 1983; Gurman, 1981; Feldman & Pinsof, 1982; Alexander & Parsons, 1982) should be read, but, just as with the purist schools, not swallowed whole. It is helpful for students to see how others have grappled with the integration of theoretical tenets, but in the final analysis, the development of ones own theory of family therapy is a very ideosyncratic and personal affair.

Liddle (1982) has suggested that therapists periodically give themselves an "ideological checkup" to allow them to explore where they stand on important theoretical issues. The theory-building learning activities presented below are used in this spirit, but with the formidable goal in mind of challenging students to carve out their own personal theory.

EXAMPLES OF THEORY BUILDING LEARNING ACTIVITIES

Triad Interviews

We typically structure a triad interview sometime toward the end of most of our theory courses. Students are put in groups of three, with each of the three students being a "focus person" for a fifteen minute period of time. During this time, the other two group members ask the focus person questions that will allow him/her to discuss basic assumptions of his/her evolving theory. This is *not* a group discussion, since only one person has the "floor" for each fifteen minute period. Students enjoy this opportunity to articulate their own opinions regarding basic theoretical questions. The following questions are shown on an overhead transparency during this exercise as possible questions for the interviewers to ask:

— How does change occur?
— What are your basic goals in therapy and how do you propose to achieve these goals?
— How is your own theory and practice of family therapy consistent or inconsistent with the theoretical models presented in this class?
— How important are the following in your own evolving theory:

—Skill building
—Affect
—Assessment (e.g., appraisal, history taking, diagnosis)
—Administrative control (structuring skills)
—Therapist-client relationship
—Enrichment
— What importance do you place on the concept of resistance? How do you deal with resistance?
— What is your theory of normative and dysfunctional family functioning?
— How do you know that change has occurred? What are your strategies for assessment?
— How do you decide who should attend therapy? (e.g., when should children, grandparents, x-spouses, etc. attend therapy and when should they be excluded?)
— To what extent do you see therapy as education?
— How much responsibility do you take for change and how much do you allow the family?
— Discuss how one or more of these constructs or principles fit or don't fit into your evolving theory: power, resistance, homeostasis, positive feedback, reinforcement, transference, behavioral rehearsal, differentiation.
— How does your therapeutic approach change across life cycle stages, ethnic groups and/or presenting problems?

Theoretical Tenet Continuum

This exercise involves designating complimentary theoretical tenets to opposite walls of the room, and then asking each student to decide on the place he/she would stand on an imaginary line between these two theoretical tenets. After everyone has decided upon his/her place, we instruct the class to get up and take that place on the continuum. Students are asked to look around them and observe their position in relation to others in the class on that quality.

This learning activity may be used in several ways. For example, we have had students discuss their choice of a position on the continuum in small groups. We have also employed selected bi-polar tenets at the beginning and end of a semester, so students can see changes in their theoretical assumptions over time. In addition, this learning activity may be used as a paper-and-pencil exercise. Another variation involves having students choose one tenet or the other (forced choice versus continuum) and then have the resulting groups debate the advantages of the theoretical tenets they chose. Such discussions are typically lively, yet the plurality of differing opinions are generally respected.

Table 1

Continuum of Selected Theoretical Tenets*

Insight is unnecessary for change to occur	Insight is necessary for change to occur
Historical information is important in understanding and changing present functioning	Historical information is unimportant in understanding and changing present functioning
Assessment is most important as an evaluation process at the beginning and end of treatment	Assessment is most important as an ongoing process within the therapy session
Interactional sequences are more relevant to therapy than organizational structure	Organizational structure is more relevant to therapy than interactional sequences
Multigenerational issues should be handled, when possible, by inviting members of the extended family into therapy	Therapy can be done with multigenerational issues just as effectively with nuclear family members only
Family member's expression of feelings can be curative and should be facilitated by the therapist	Expressions of feelings often inhibit change and should be blocked by the therapist
The therapist should be a model of clear, direct communication	The therapist is most helpful when he/she speaks indirectly and metaphorically
Problematic behavior is maintained by the family's homeostatic (morphostatic, negative feedback) processes	Problematic behavior is maintained by the family's ineffective attempts to change (morphagenesis, positive feedback)
The client is responsible for change	The therapist is responsible for change
The therapist's actions during a session are best if planned	The therapist's actions during a session are best if spontaneous
The overall goal of therapy is client growth	The overall goal of therapy is problem resolution
Significant change occurs between the therapy sessions	Significant change occurs within the therapy sessions

*We are indebted to Dr. Janine Roberts, University of Massachusettes-Amherst, and Mr. Mark Hirschmann, Purdue University, for the initial version of many of these bi-polar items.

Supervision Worksheets

In our course in Family Therapy Supervision, each student must develop a supervision worksheet to aid him/her in providing live and/or indirect supervision to family therapists. Supervisors-in-training are encouraged to develop forms that will help supervisees bridge their own theory with what they actually do in therapy. Consquently, supervisors-in-training are learning to help their own supervisee think through theoretical suppositions and how these suppositions might be translated into therapy goals and strategies. An example of such a worksheet is included in Appendix A.

Personal Theory Paper and Videotape Presentation

Each family therapy student completes a unique specialization preliminary examination at Purdue toward the end of his/her doctoral program. This prelim includes the writing of a thirty-page personal theory of family therapy paper, the demonstration of this theory in selected videotaped segments of actual therapy sessions, and the formal presentation of this theory and videotape to students and faculty.

The integrative personal theory paper details the student's personal approach to family therapy, and includes the following sections: a) basic conceptualization of the family as a social system, b) views concerning pathology and health in family systems, c) goals of therapy, d) the process of change, e) intervention strategies, and f) implications of the approach for research. This paper is intended to provide the student with an opportunity to compare and contrast his/her theoretical assumptions with those of major theorists. As such, the paper represents a creative expression of the student's own views as he/she dialogues with the key documents in the field. Faculty and other MFT students are expected to read the paper prior to the presentation so that it can be a time for dialogue with the presenter.

The formal theory presentation in which the videotaped therapy segments are shown lasts approximately 90 minutes. During the initial ten minutes, the student gives an uninterrupted overview of the interventions that will subsquently be presented in the videotape and indicates how, in a very general sense, they are consistent with his/her theory as articulated in the paper. Following this introduction, the student presents the videotape and discusses the interventions, with the primary focus being on the interventions themselves rather than on family dynamics or family problems. The student shows how these specific interventions are consistent with his/her personal theory and demonstrates how they are effective in achieving their assumed goals. Apart from the ten minute introduction and the first ten minutes of the tape, anyone can ask questions at any time. The mood of these presentations is generally supportive and respectful, and questions typically stretch the student to articulate and defend his/her personal theory in what amounts to a formalized rite of passage.

Other Learning Activities

We have discussed other theory-building learning activities elsewhere (Piercy & Sprenkle, 1984). For example, such learning activities as dyad discussions, simulation papers, position papers, reaction papers, and journal days may be used to involve students in examining, criticizing, and integrating various theoretical tenets.

CONCLUSION

The key figures of family therapy were revolutionaries. They took strong, often unpopular, theoretical stands that ran counter to the Zeitgeist of their time and that paved the way for the theoretical models taught today. We believe that a current frontier in family therapy involves the task of taking the best of these models and integrating them in ways that are sensitive to various therapist styles, life cycle stages, family dynamics, and presenting problems. Graduate family therapy education, therefore, must develop bold and creative procedures to help future family therapists with the formidable process of informed and critical theory integration. The present paper represents an initial attempt to explicate this need and includes illustrative ways that family therapy educators might begin addressing the process of family therapy theory building.

REFERENCES

Alexander, J. & Parsons, B. (1982) *Functional family therapy.* Monterey, CA: Brooks/Cole.

Allred, G. & Kersey, F. (1977). The AIAC, a design for systematically analyzing marriage and family counselors: A progress report. *Journal of Marriage and Family Counseling, 3,* 17-26.

Bowen, M. (1978). *Family therapy in clinical practice.* New York: Aronson.

Cleghorn, J. & Levin, S. (1973). Training family therapists by setting learning objectives. *American Journal of Orthopsychiatry, 43* 439-446.

Constantine, J., Stone-Fish, L. & Piercy, F. (1984). A systematic procedure for teaching positive connotation. *Journal of Marital and Family Therapy, 10*(3), 313-316.

Duhl, B.S. (1983). *From the inside out and other metaphors.* New York: Brunner/Mazel.

Duhl, B.S. & Duhl, F.J. (1981). Integrative family therapy. In A.S. Gurman & D.P. Kniskern (Eds.), *Handbook of family therapy. New York: Brunner/Mazel.*

Falicov, C., Constantine, J. & Breunlin, D. (1981). Teaching family therapy: A program based on learning objectives. *Journal of Marital and Family Therapy, 7,* 497-506.

Feldman, L.B. & Pinsof, W.M. (1982). Problem maintenance in family systems: An integrative model. *Journal of Marital and Family Therapy, 8,* 295-308.

Fraser, S. (1982). Structural and strategic family therapy: A basis for marriage or grounds for divorce? *Journal of Marital and Family Therapy, 8*(2).

Garrigan, J. & Bambrick, A. (1977). Introducing novice family therapists to "go-between" techniques of family therapy. *Family Process, 16,* 237-246.

Gurman, A.S. (1981). Integrative marital therapy: Toward the development of an interpersonal approach. In S. Budman (Ed.), *Forms of brief therapy.* New York: Guilford.

Kaslow, F. & Associates (1977). *Supervision consultation, and staff training in the helping professions.* San Francisco: Jossey-Bass.

Kniskern, D. & Gurman, A. (1979). Research on training in marriage and family therapy: Status, issues, and directions. *Journal of Marital and Family Therapy, 5,* 83-94.

Lebow, J.L. (1984). On the value of integrating approaches to family therapy. *Journal of Marital and Family Therapy, 10*(2), 127-138.

Liddle, H.A. (1980). On teaching a contextual of systemic therapy: Training content, goals, and methods. *American Journal of Family Therapy, 8*(1), 58-69.

Liddle, H. (1982a). Family therapy training: Current issues, future trends. *International Journal of Family Therapy, 4*(2), 81-97.

Liddle, H.A. (1982b). On the problems of eclectism: A call for epistemological clarification and human scale theories. *Family Process, 21,* 243-250.

Liddle, H.A. & Halpin, R. (1978). Family therapy training and supervision literature: A comparative review. *Journal of Marriage and Family Counseling, 4,* 77-98.

Liddle, H.A. & Saba, G.W. (1982). On teaching family therapy at the introductory level: A conceptual model emphasizing a pattern which connects training and therapy. *Journal of Marital and Family Therapy, 8*(1), 63-73.

Liddle, H.A. & Schwartz, R.C. (1983). Live supervision/consultation: Conceptual and pragmatic guidelines for family therapy trainees. *Family Process, 22*(4), 477-490.

Mohammed, A. & Piercy, F. (1983). The effects of two methods of training and sequencing on structuring and relationship skills of family therapists. *American Journal of Family Therapy, 11*(4), 64-71.

Nichols, W. (1979). Education of marriage and family therapists: Some trends and implications. *Journal of Marital and Family Therapy, 5,* 19-28.

Piercy, F. (1984). The true believer and eclectic. *Family Therapy Networker,* January-February, 21.

Piercy, F., Laird, R. & Mohammad, Z. (1983). A family therapist rating scale. *Journal of Marital and Family Therapy, 9,* 49-59.

Piercy, F. & Sprenkle, D. (1983). Ethical, legal and professional issues in family therapy: A graduate level course. *Journal of Marital and Family Therapy, 9*(4), 393-401.

Piercy, F. & Sprenkle, D. (1984). The process of family therapy education. *Journal of Marital and Family Therapy.*

Pinsof, W.M. (1983). Integrative problem-centered therapy: Toward the synthesis of family and individual psychotherapies. *Journal of Marital and Family Therapy, 9,* 19-35.

Pittman, F. (1983). Of cults and superstars. *Family Therapy Networker, 7*(1), 28-29.

Sluzki, C.E. (1983). Process structure and world views: Toward an integrated view of systemic models in family therapy. *Family Process 22*(4), 469-477.

Sprenkle, D. & Piercy, F. (1984). Research in family therapy: A graduate level course. *Journal of Marital and Family Therapy, 10*(3), 225-240.

Stanton, M.D. (1981). An integrated structural/strategic approach to family therapy. *Journal of Marital and Family Therapy, 7,* 427-440.

Tomm, K. & Wright, L. (1979). Training in family therapy: Perceptual, conceptual, and executive skills. *Family Process, 18,* 227-250.

Winkle, W., Piercy, F. & Hovestadt, A. (1981). A marriage and family therapy curriculum. *Journal of Marital and Family Therapy, 7,* 201-210.

Appendix A

WORKSHEET FOR PLANNING AND REVIEWING SESSION STRATEGIES*

Therapist_____   Supervisor_____

_____
(Therapist completes this section before the therapy session)

Date_____   Client ID_____   Session#_____

Theoretical Approach:

Long-term goal. What do you want to happen in this family, or couple, before therapy is completed?

Appendix A continued

Session goal. What do you want to happen in the family, or couple, in this session?

Strategy for this session. Circle one or two strategies below to designate the primary plans for this session. For each strategy, indicate specifically what is to be accomplished. (You may use the back to plan how to carry out these strategies.)

Provide a certain experience   Modify family structure

Teach ideas   Interrupt behavioral sequence

Teach skills   Provide information

Have clients discuss certain ideas   Assign homework

Other strategies:

_____

*Therapist completes this section with the supervisor after the session (preferably, during videotaped supervision of the session)

Was the planned strategy executed? If so, what specific interventions contributed to that execution? If not, why not?

How well was the session goal accomplished? Discuss the fit of the session goal with the clients' presenting problems and the effectiveness of the strategies for accomplishing the goal.
_____
*Adapted from a worksheet developed by John H. Lasley, Purdue University, 1984.

Family Therapy Supervision:
An Introduction and Consumer's Guide

W. Robert Beavers

ABSTRACT. Supervision in family therapy is becoming more theoretically homogeneous, with a definite systems orientation. In this paper, family therapy supervision is introduced in relation to its predecessor, individual psychotherapy supervision. In addition, strengths and weaknesses of various settings where family supervision takes place (i.e., universities, private practices, free-standing institutes, public agencies, and short-term workshops) are discussed. Finally, some of the rules and expectations of the Commission on Supervision of the American Association for Marriage and Family Therapy, developed during the writer's tenure on this body, are presented.

Supervision in marriage and family therapy is both a legitimate offspring of individual psychotherapy supervision and a mutant, representing qualitative differences from the parent. The history of psychotherapy is a continuous record of the apprenticeship method of learning a trade (i.e., the experienced master directs the novice in the activities of this trade). Often the service or product is paid for as if it had come from the master.

Individual psychotherapy generally maintained this apprenticeship model. The most intricate elaboration of this model is reflected in psychoanalytic training, in which institutes grant approval to individuals after years of analysis and carefully supervised therapy experience.

The "mutation" aspect of family therapy supervision refers to the opening up of what the master does, to be seen directly by the apprentice, and the observation of what the apprentice is doing, with immediate interaction of supervisor, therapist, trainees, and clients, each in a position to influence the other (Kempster and Savitsky, 1967; Olson and Pegg, 1979; Glick and Kessler, 1980). This dramatic alteration was due to several factors working in concert. First, in family therapy, there was a near violent reaction against the concepts and practices of psychoanalysts (though some of these came to be repeated in family therapy supervision, as will be noted later). Second, there is much more of a "psychodrama" quality

---

W. Robert Beavers, M.D., is Clinical Director of the Southwest Family Institute, and Clinical Professor of Psychiatry, University of Texas Health Science Center, Dallas, Texas. Dr. Beavers is also President-Elect of the American Association for Marriage and Family Therapy. His mailing address is 3613 Cedar Springs Road, Dallas, TX 75219.

to family therapy that cries for an audience. (It is instructive that at least three notable family therapists at an outstanding family training institute were or are married to Broadway producers!)

Third, the change in emphasis from cognition to interaction all but necessitated visual instruction and family observation. Fourth, the technical advances in video equipment have made it increasingly easy for family therapy to be viewed in addition to being talked about. It is simple to add verbal communication to observation with either video equipment or one-way mirror (Whiffen and Byng Hall, 1982).

Being a veteran psychiatrist, I was trained in the old style of presenting process notes and being critiqued at a safe distance from patients. I learned family work by doing it, on the sly, using one-way mirror and audiotapes to develop and maintain contact with peers who were interested in the relationship of family patterns to individual psychiatric symptoms. As a resident psychiatrist, I learned to distinguish between two kinds of supervisors: those who expected me to treat the patients and use their supervision for skill enhancement, and those who used me as an instrument to treat the patient. The latter supervisors expected me to learn by doing what I was told. The two distinctions are still valuable in understanding variations in family therapy supervision (Henley and Weber, 1983).

A second distinction is useful in understanding family therapy supervision: the master may help in *managing* a client or family situation, and s/he may help in developing technical *skills* and strategies. Both of these are important and both have limitations (Montalvo, 1973). For mental health professionals who are learning family therapy, the emphasis reasonably should be on developing techniques. Fledgling therapists new in the field need more help in understanding family patterns, developing requisite skills, and establishing overall case management and treatment goals.

A third important distinction regarding family therapy supervision is that of individual versus group. Early in the family therapy movement, sion, modeled after analytic supervision, was the usual a systemic theoretical model evolved and with the use of and video machinery, group supervision has become more popular. There is some conflict regarding the val- versus group supervision. This conflict often is more oretical. Supervisors in private practice and small agen- dividual supervision more feasible—the apprenticeship faithfully, fits their situation. On the other hand, an amber of family therapy training institutes, with skilled chers collaborating to provide a program of training, effective to have group supervision. Such supervision often involves the use of one-way mirrors and immediate supervisory input by way of telephone call-ins, mid- and end-of-session conferences, etc. (In order to become acquainted with the wide variety of supervisory procedures, see the annotated bibliography of training literature at the end of this issue.)

This conflict is sharper because the American Association for Marriage and Family Therapy (AAMFT), the largest organization of family therapy and the most active in establishing standards in the field, requires 200 hours of supervision, of which 100 of these must be individual supervision. Many free standing institutes consider this latter requirement onerous and unnecessary, but veteran individual supervisors believe it to be vital.

My own belief, from the vantage point of the initial Chairman of the Commission on Supervision of AAMFT, is that the importance of trainee qualifications has been too little appreciated in this controversy. Seasoned mental health professionals who receive training in family therapy already have a professional identity, role models for ethical conduct, and experience in case management. They can utilize group supervision best, with its emphasis on transmitting techniques and treatment strategies. However, there are ever larger numbers of novice therapists seeking family therapy training who have no other professional identity. They must be socialized as mental health professionals while also receiving specific technical training in family therapy; individual supervision with its apprenticeship strengths is most valuable for this group.

THEORETICAL ORIENTATION

Currently, family therapy supervision is a potpourri of many varied theoretical underpinnings. There are supervisors who identify themselves primarily with psychoanalytic concepts, Gestalt theory, transactional analysis, behaviorism, communication theory, and (more and more) family systems theory. Family systems theory, however, is becoming the standard basic conceptual framework for the field, even though its definition remains varied and perhaps murky. The AAMFT brochure on the approved supervisor offers a decent working definition of marriage and family therapy illustrating the emerging consensus of a systems orientation as the basis of practice *and of supervision:*

"The clinical practice of marriage and family therapy is:
   a) Understood to be face-to-face sessions with the clients usually in periods of approximately one hour each;
   b) Sustained and intense, and as indicated by the needs of the clients;
   c) Considered usually to involve a couple or a whole family. Marriage and Family Therapy (MFT) is distinctly different from group therapy, family life education, marital enrichment, expanding

human potential, and/or other group procedures. The AAMFT recognizes the value of these other procedures and that some marriage and family therapists occasionally may use them. However, the AAMFT does not consider these procedures to be the clinical practice of marriage and family therapy;

d) Understood to deal primarily with relationships, interpersonal interaction, and systems theory. MFT thereby requires special conceptualization as well as procedures which are distinct from the individually oriented therapies. Historically, individually-oriented therapists sometimes develop the special skills of MFT which is a distinctly different procedure. Many marriage and family therapists have experience in both areas. It is the specific expertise in interpersonal relationships, interaction, and systems theory, however, which qualifies a professional as a marriage and family therapist.'' (American Association for Marriage and Family Therapy, 1983)

Supervision of family therapy treatment is to be distinguished from treatment, from administrative supervision, from cotherapy, and from discussion of cases with peers. It can be defined as the training of professionals by more experienced clinicians/teacher in the clinical specialty of marriage and family therapy. It is not treatment of the trainee, since the focus is on the healing of a troubled marriage or family; any legitimate discussion of the supervisee's weak spots will be in the context of his or her clinical endeavor. Any discussion of administrative problems or decisions must be secondary to and directly pertinent to treatment strategies. There may be occasional times of sitting in a treatment session with a supervisee, in order to supervise more effectively, but this is quite apart from being a co-therapist.

Candidates for Approved Supervisor (a designation from the Commission on Supervision of AAMFT) are expected to have a systemic orientation as exhibited by such concepts as: 1) Symptoms have meaning to families as well as individuals, 2) Individual emotional illness can be effectively altered by changing the patterns of the person's immediate family or network, 3) Multiple levels of human existence are important in illness and health, and each level impacts the other (e.g., a couple's conflict can influence the severity of a child's asthma and vice versa); 4) there are reverberating levels in intervention that influence each other (e.g., the supervisor/trainee interaction may influence the therapist/family interface and vice versa), 5) The vice versas in 3 and 4 suggest the importance of circularity, i.e., causes can be effects, and effects can be causes. This is in sharp contrast to linear or simple one-way concepts of symptom production.

These concepts are reasonably precise and communicable and do not exhaust or limit the varied theoretical conceptualizations possible within a systems orientation.

THE STRENGTHS AND WEAKNESSES
OF SUPERVISION ENVIRONMENTS:
A CONSUMER'S GUIDE

There are five areas in which most family therapy supervision takes place: a) in universities training marital and family therapists, b) in private practice, c) in free-standing family institutes, d) in agencies primarily serving the community's mental health needs, and e) in time-limited workshops. There are special possibilities in each of these areas, and special risks of poor quality supervision of which potential supervisees should be aware. I will attempt to be something of a Ralph Nader of the supervisory process in describing these possibilities and potential problems. My "consumer report" will be written in broad strokes to reflect my own general opinions regarding certain tendencies of supervision environments. Exceptions, of course, will exist in each case.

University Settings

Supervisors in a university are often less hurried, quite conscientious, and thoroughly theoretically grounded in the latest systemic orientations. These supervisors are likely to teach a variety of theoretical models, both through academic coursework and through supervision, and are typically more disposed to theoretical integration than to indoctrination. Their supervisees can expect time and individual attention from them, and most universities have better than average facilities for training. There are potential problems, however. The supervisor may have only a few thousand hours of clinical experience and may be more competent in theory than in the "street savvy" that marks a clinician who has been full time in clinical practice for many years. A further problem in many of the university settings might be the rather narrow and limited clinical population (Berg, 1978), typically young and bright couples enrolled in graduate studies who come to the university treatment facility. This is a significant drawback; no matter how skilled the supervisor, the material is the ultimate teacher. Families with a schizophrenic teenager, with a father who has manic episodes, with a retarded thirty-year-old son, with an aged parent who becomes unable to care for him/herself—all these provide an overwhelming impact on trainees that, when mastered, develops therapeutic confidence to a far greater degree than experience in a program that primarily deals with marital conflict and undisciplined small children. Wise academic professionals realize this, of course, and struggle to provide their students with clinical facilities that will offer material to challenge them and supervisors capable of helping master these challenges.

Private Practice

Still an important source of family therapy supervision, private practice is now less significant than in the past. Again there are historical parallels with the psychoanalytic; family therapy, like psychoanalysis, was initially shunned by academia and flourished in a kind of private practice underground with individual zealots providing the steam for the new movement. As respectability embraces family therapy, establishment organizations move in to co-opt the previously revolutionary concepts and activities.

From supervisors in private practice, a potential supervisee should expect clinical competence and a burning desire to communicate this competence. Private practice has all the virtues and vices of capitalism; the fittest (as defined by the marketplace) survive, and if a trainee plans to risk that marketplace, a private practitioner is extremely useful as a role model. If that private practitioner can and does, in some way, share the richness of his/her caseload, we have the traditional strengths of the apprenticeship model—a young person dealing with highly varied clinical problems under close supervision of an experienced, competent professional.

The downside of this category of supervisory experience is primarily related to *time*. It takes time to supervise, and the needs of supervisees frequently do not fit into the contracted session time. Private practice seldom provides casual, unstructured opportunities for discussion. There is also the problem of clinical material; often the private practitioner does not find it practical to share the clients coming in his or her door, but rather expects the supervisee to round up his/her own clients, an excellent arrangement for established professionals, but a real problem for the novice.

Further, the tempo of private practice is often not conducive to experimentation in supervision. Innovations such as group planning of family prescriptions or frequent telephone contact between supervisor and supervisee (Gershenson and Cohen, 1978, Whiffen and Byng-Hall, 1982), are unusual in private practice. Innovation requires time and a sense of play that is uncharacteristic of the busy marketplace.

Family Therapy Institutes

Innovation and experimentation in clinical techniques and strategies are common in free-standing (non-university affiliated) training institutes.

Here many private practitioners can "cut loose" with their interests in theory and their desire for inefficient (i.e., joyful) training work. Two of the oldest, the Ackerman Institute in New York City and the Mental Research Institute in Palo Alto, still have leadership roles, while scores of others have developed around the nation.

Supervision in these institutes can be rich and intense; senior clinicians usually teach as a labor of love rather than as an academic duty. With the innovative tendency, institute experience can give the trainee a sense of being on the cutting edge of the field. Hands-on work with families under live supervision and a watching group of peers provide stressful but powerful learning opportunity (Gershenson and Cohen, 1978).

Institutes usually have been founded, however, to promote a particular treatment approach. They are likely to be technique focused rather than being as theoretically broad as are good academic institutions. Supervisees can acquire a false sense of superiority as clinicians when they have actually become adept at only one of many potentially valuable methods for inducing change in families (Olson and Pegg, 1979). In this, I see a faithful recreation of the analytic institutes so vigorously attacked by the founders of some of the outstanding family therapy training facilities. Many of these founders, such as Don Jackson, Nathan Ackerman, and Salvador Minuchin, had analytic training. Though many of the concepts were abandoned, the attitude of training through indoctrination of theory and practice remains.

Public Service Agencies

This source of supervision is more a potential one than a current reality, since traditional concepts of the mental health professional's roles and duties have made it slow and hard to introduce a family treatment model to public mental health facilities. Resistance to the approach, and resistance to the hiring of family therapists have meant a paucity of good training opportunities in public agencies.

However, as the cost effectiveness of family treatment is becoming more evident, and expenditures on mental health continue to rise, "the times they are a-changin'". A first evidence of this is the increased number of applications for Approved Supervisor status from mental health professionals working in public agencies, who are relatively untrained and unskilled in family therapy. Agency administrators understandably find it simpler and much cheaper for family therapy trainees involved in practice or internship in their agencies to be supervised by presently employed professionals. A second and brighter evidence of change is the number of professionals in public agencies who are obtaining special training in marital and family therapy, often with support from employers.

The trainee will usually find a wide variety of clinical material and people seriously in need of help in these public agencies. With adequate supervision, veterans of this training can well consider themselves battle-tested and superior mental health professionals. They may, however, risk being used to meet a never-ending demand for services with too little and inadequate case supervision. Supervision may, in these settings, be so loosely defined as to be little more than discussion of administrative problems.

Workshops

Many students and practitioners attempt to increase their skills through workshops on family therapy techniques that are focused and time limited. These workshops provide an opportunity to learn from prominent clinicians/teachers who demonstrate their methods and, in some situations, supervise therapists' work with the goal of developing expertise in novel treatment techniques. While useful as augmentation of marital and family therapy training, these workshops should not be considered by trainees or sponsoring institutions as a primary means of training professionals. Supervision requires constancy of therapist with clients and supervisor with therapist.

SUPERVISION OF SUPERVISION

The task of defining adequate supervisors in marital and family therapy was accepted by AAMFT in 1971, with the establishment of a committee on supervision to perform this function. In 1983, this committee was converted to the Commission on Supervision, a semi-autonomous body that serves the field of family therapy, much as the AAMFT Commission on Accreditation, by establishing standards and evaluating performance of training institutions, serves the United States and Canada in addition to the AAMFT. The latest AAMFT guidebook for the Approved Supervisor (AAMFT, 1983) states:

A candidate for designation as an AAMFT Approved Supervisor may follow one of two alternative tracks:
  a) Track 1

  1. Has been in clinical practice as a marriage and family therapist at least five (5) years;
  2. Has at least two (2) years' experience supervising MFT:
  3. Has received at least 36 hours of individual supervision of his/her supervision of MFT of at least two (2) supervisees who meet mini-

mum qualifications for Student or Associate in AAMFT. This is usually for a period of one year and shall not exceed two years. Customarily, supervision of supervision is scheduled once a week; once every other week is considered minimum. Up to 18 hours of this individual supervision may be earned through group supervision at the ratio of three (3) hours of group supervision to one (1) hour of individual supervision. Thus, a maximum of 54 hours of group supervision of supervision may replace 18 hours of individual supervision. Group size shall not exceed six (6) candidates. The candidate for appointment as an Approved Supervisor must complete the training for supervision with an AAMFT Approved Supervisor. Supervision of supervision of two (2) people conjointly may be counted as individual; and,

4. Attendance and participation at a workshop on supervision issues, presented by the Commission on Supervision, at an annual AAMFT conference, is required for non-AAMFT members.

b) Track II

The Commission on Supervision retains the authority to approve as an Approved Supervisor persons of prominence in the MFT field. Such prominence will be indicate by:

1. At least 10 years of experience in specialized therapy and supervision within the MFT field;
2. Written documentation of a systemic orientation in any published materials and in the written materials provided to the Commission in support of the application;
3. Prominence in one's community or the nation as an educator/trainer in MFT;
4. Letters of recommendation from two AAMFT Approved Supervisors who are able to attest to the candidate's competence in the supervision of MFT trainees and to the candidate's adherence to a systemic orientation and prominence in the field; and,
5. Attendance and participation at a workshop on supervision issues, presented by the Commission on Supervision, at an annual AAMFT conference, is required for non-AAMFT members.

Thus it is possible to be an AAMFT Approved Supervisor but not be a member of AAMFT. Such occurrences are rare, however, as most professionals who are active in the field and desire the Approved Supervisor status wish to belong to the preeminent organization that represents the field. For some professionals, this designation is seen more as an advantage to their trainees than to them. Approving those experienced profes-

sionals expands the opportunities for many clinicians to achieve membership in AAMFT.

CONCLUSION

Supervision in family therapy is becoming more clearly defined with a
systems orientation. As the field develops, more competent supervision in
a variety of clinical and educational settings is available. The guidelines
of the Commission on Supervision of the American Association for Marriage and Family Therapy are becoming the standards for this clinical activity.

REFERENCES

American Association for Marriage and Family Therapy (1983). Brochure, The Approved
    Supervisor, Washington, D.C.
Berg, B. (1978). Learning family therapy through simulation. *Psychotherapy: Theory, research
    and practice,* Spring, 56-64.
Glick, I. D. and Kessler, V. R. (1980). Training for the family therapist. In I. D. Glick and V. R.
    Kessler (Eds.), *Marital and family therapy,* New York: Grune and Stratton.
Gershenson, J., and Cohen, M. (1978). Direct open supervision: A team approach. *Family Process,*
    17, 225-230.
Henley, R., and Weber, K. (1983). Training in marriage and family therapy. In B. Wolman and
    G. Stricker (Eds.), *Handbook for family and marital therapy.* New York: Plenum Press.
Kempster, S. A., & Savitsky, E. (1967). Training family therapists through 'Live' supervision.
    In N. W. Ackerman, F. L. Beatman, and J. N. Sherman (Eds.), *Expanding theory and practice
    family therapy,* 125-134, New York: Family Service Association.
Montalvo, B. (1973). Aspects of live supervision. *Family Process, 12,* 343-359.
Olson, V. J. & Pegg, P. F. (1979). Through the looking glass: The experiences of two family
    therapy trainees with live supervision. *Family Process, 18,* 463-469.
Whiffen, R., & Byng-Hall, J. (1982). *Family therapy supervision.* London: Academic Press.

Family Therapy as a Profession or Professional Specialty: Implications for Training*

David L. Fenell
Alan J. Hovestadt

ABSTRACT. A three-level model for integrating family therapy training into graduate education is presented. This model proposes training programs for family therapy education at the (a) professional level, (b) professional specialty level and (c) elective level of study. Discussed are implications and considerations for beginning family therapy training programs at each of these levels.

Family therapy generally is thought to have had its beginnings in the early 1950s. During this time, pioneers in the field began seeing families conjointly to help alleviate the symptoms of one of the family members. Many of the pioneers were psychiatrists and psychologists specializing in the treatment of psychotic children. Early pioneers such as John Bell, Nathan Ackerman, Theodore Lidz, Lyman Wynne, Murray Bowen, and Carl Whitaker were laying a part of the foundation for the profession of family therapy that was to emerge in the 1970s (Broderick & Schrader, 1981).

FAMILY THERAPY AS A PROFESSION

The issue of whether or not family therapy is a profession is loaded with controversy (Gurman and Kniskern, 1981). We believe that family therapy merits the status of a profession because it meets most of the established criteria of a profession.

Broderick (1981) states that three criteria define a profession. These are (a) self-awareness of the profession and the identification of a body of

*The preparation of this manuscript was supported in part by NIMH Grant MH 16608.

David L. Fenell, Ph.D., is an Assistant Professor of Guidance and Counseling, School of Education, Austin Bluffs Parkway, University of Colorado at Colorado Springs, CO 80907.

Alan J. Hovestadt, Ed.D., is Professor of Counseling Psychology and Chair, Department of Counseling and Personnel, Western Michigan University, Kalamazoo, MI 49008.

experts, (b) a set of skills, techniques and theories requiring advanced training with established standards of performance, and (c) a recognition of this body of experts and the usefulness of their expert service by the larger society.

Similarly, Burr and Leigh (1983) list seven criteria for the establishment of a discipline: (a) the existence of a unique subject matter, (b) the existence of an adequate body of theory and research, (c) the existence of a unique methodology, (d) the existence of support structures such as professional associations, professional journals, and universities with academic departments, (e) demonstrated utility to society, (f) the existence of a community of scholars to teach the discipline and guide research, and (g) a belief that the profession exists.

Since most of these criteria (perhaps with the exception of the existence of a unique methodology) are met by family therapy, it may legitimately be considered a profession. The maturity of family therapy (Burr and Leigh, 1983) together with its rapidly increasing body of research and theory (Olson, Russell, and Sprenkle, 1980) represent a strong case for its identification as a separate profession distinct from other mental health care professions. Additionally, the Office of U.S. Secretary of Education in the U.S. Department of Education officially recognizes family therapy as a profession. Also, ten states have granted statutory recognition for professionals demonstrating appropriate training and skills in marriage and family therapy (Johnson, 1984).

The recognition of family therapy as a profession by the larger society it serves is directly related to the profession's ability to attain legitimacy and power. For family therapy to gain this legitimacy and power, high quality professional graduate training is a necessity. To the extent that graduate family therapy training programs produce top quality therapists who maintain their professional identity as "family therapists," the profession will receive increasing recognitions by the larger society and will gain further legitimacy and power.

FAMILY THERAPY AS A PROFESSIONAL SPECIALTY

While family therapy meets most of the criteria for recognition as a distinct profession, this proposition does not receive universal support. At the present time, family therapy is being taught as a professional specialty in a variety of departments in institutions of higher education throughout the United States and Canada. Family therapy, for example, is taught as a professional specialty in departments of psychiatry, psychology, social work, nursing, professional counseling, and clinical pastoral education. In each of these departments, the primary education and socialization of the students is in the profession identified by the department name. Thus, students studying family therapy in a department of psychology are primarily trained and socialized as psychologists and secondarily trained in family therapy.

This situation highlights a potential conflict area in the definition of family therapy. Is family therapy a profession or a specialization area belonging within an older, and more established profession? Can it be both?

Programs that propose to train family therapists must make explicit whatever definition of family therapy is decided upon to all who participate in the training program. If this clear definitional statement is not determined and interpreted to faculty, administrators and students, it is likely that family therapy training goals and objectives will conflict with previously established departmental goals and objectives. Cooper and Charnofsky (1983) and Liddle and Halpin (1978) point out that intradepartmental problems may arise from theoretical differences that exist between faculty that adhere to an intrapsychic model of behavior change and faculty that conceptualize from systems-based family therapy models of change.

THE TRAINING MODEL

In this chapter, a three-level training model is described for the preparation of family therapists. This model is based on a previous paper (Hovestadt, Fenell and Piercy, 1983) and proposes a conceptual framework to meet the needs of graduate university training programs offering family therapy as either a profession, professional specialty or area for elective study.

Level One: Family Therapy Degree or Degree-Equivalent

A Level-One training program recognizes family therapy as a mental health profession offered in a department that awards a corresponding degree or degree-equivalent. This level of training is appropriate in institutions that define family therapy as a distinct profession. The degree-equivalent family therapy training program is defined as a program offering comprehensive family therapy training on a co-equal basis with the parent profession in a department that awards a degree other than one titled marriage and/or family therapy. The degree equivalent program, in all other respects, meets nationally established family therapy curricular requirements stated in the *Marriage and Family Therapy: Manual on Accreditation,* (1981). Examples of Level-One programs occur in Departments of Child Development and Family Studies, Psychology, Sociology, Social Work, and Counseling and Guidance.

Level-One Curriculum. The Level-One degree or degree-equivalent program in family therapy is specified within a model curriculum developed by the Commission on Accreditation for Marriage and Family Therapy Education. A comprehensive marriage and family therapy curriculum at either the master's or doctoral level will contain all components of this model. The components of the curriculum are reported in Table 1 *(Marriage and Family Therapy: Manual on Accreditation,* 1981).

The Marital and Family Systems area of study develops a fundamental introduction to the systems approach to therapeutic intervention. The student learns to think in systemic terms and conceptualize family interaction at multiple system levels. The study of family development also is considered an important component of the family therapist's education. Also included in this area of study should be the nuclear family, its numerous derivatives and family-of-origin theory.

The Marital and Family Therapy area of study is expected to produce a comprehensive knowledge of the major theories of system change, as well as the therapeutic practices evolving from each of the theories. Theories examined in this content area may include (a) strategic, (b) structural, (c) communications, (d) behavioral, (e) experiential, and (f) object relations.

Study in the area of Individual Development is included to provide knowledge of normal and abnormal individual personality development. Courses offered may include: (a) human development, (b) personality theory, (c) behavior pathology, and (d) human sexuality.

The Professional Studies area is designed to contribute to the professional development and socialization of the family therapist. This area of study assists the student in the development of professional attitude and identity. Course content may include (a) the role of family therapist, (b) licensure and credentialing issues in family therapy, (c) professional ethics and family law, and (d) information that may be of use in establishing an independent practice as a family therapist.

The Research area of study at Level-One is designed to prepare family therapists to read knowledgeably in psychotherapy and family therapy and includes information focusing on research design and statistics. The required research course at Level-One maintains a primary focus on research in family therapy and family studies.

The Supervised Clinical Practice area of training requires a substantial practicum/internship providing students with therapy experience with couples, families, and individuals. This clinical experience should be supervised by appropriately qualified family therapists. (This area of study is described in more detail in the next section of this chapter.)

The Electives selected by students in a Level-One training program frequently are designed to add depth to their study of marriage and family therapy. Frequently, these courses include more specific study of one or more of the systems theories presented in the required coursework.

Table 1
Model Curriculum

Area of Study		Sem Hrs	Qtr Hrs
1. Marital and Family Systems	2–4 courses	6–12*	8–16**
2. Marital and Family Therapy	2–4 courses	6–12*	8–16**
3. Individual Development	2–4 courses	6–12*	8–16**
4. Professional Studies	1 course	3	4
5. Research	1 course	3	4
6. Supervised Clinical Practice	1 year	9	12
7. Electives	1 course	3	4
		45	60

* 27 Hr. Minimum in total of areas 1, 2, 3.
** 36 Hr. Minimum in total of areas 1, 2, 3.
(from Marriage and Family Therapy: Manual on Accreditation, 1981)

To plan and implement a Level-One training program that includes each of the seven areas described, it may be necessary to coordinate course offerings from several departments within an academic institution (Piercy & Hovestadt, 1980).

Level-One Supervised Clinical Training. The Level-One training program requires a supervised clinical experience in family therapy with couples and families for eight to ten hours per week. This experience should continue for a minimum of one and one-half years. A minimum of 500 hours of direct client contact is expected to be achieved during this period. It is recommended that the supervisors of the family therapy clinical experience be Approved Supervisors in the American Association for Marriage and Family Therapy, or equivalently prepared individuals. The student's case load should include a variety of cases composed of work with individuals, couples, and families representing a wide range of presenting problems. Both individual and group supervision of these cases should be provided. Training and supervision for students in Level-One programs usually take place in university sponsored and operated family therapy training centers during the initial phases of clinical skill development. A schematic depicting one approach to sequencing family therapy coursework and supervised clinical experience is shown in Figure 1 (From Piercy, Hovestadt, Fenell, Franklin, and McKeon, 1982).

Considerations. Level-One training is most easily implemented by programs that define family therapy as a distinct profession and offer a degree in marriage and family therapy.

Programs that define family therapy as a degree *equivalent* and seek to establish a Level-One program should be aware of certain problems that may arise in implementing and sustaining this level of training. Several Level-One family therapy training programs established within mental health disciplines other than marriage and family therapy have been accredited by the Commission on Accreditation of the American Association for Marriage and Family Therapy. The number of AAMFT accredited graduate training programs now number sixteen (Johnson, 1984), and graduate students appear eager to enter such programs (Thomas, 1983). When students apply for admission to these professional programs, it is important that they be informed that coursework specifically related to the parent profession is required in addition to the family therapy training sequence. If this information is not spelled out clearly, disappointment may develop among students who selected the department specifically for the family therapy component of the training program.

After a degree-equivalent program has been established and is operational, it may become apparent that some faculty and students are more excited by the concepts, literature, and professional associations of family therapy than by the concepts, literature and professional associations of

Figure 1.

Model for Sequencing Family Therapist Training

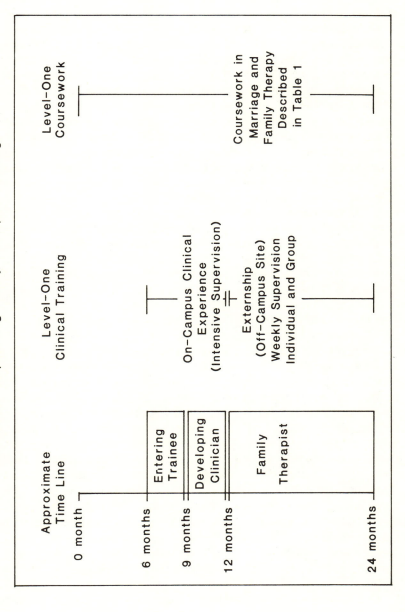

the parent department. This is especially true if the family therapy training program is the primary factor that attracted the students to the department.

Departments that successfully sustain Level-One family therapy training programs at the professional degree-equivalent level are those that have a secure faculty who are not threatened by the ideas presented by faculty and students involved in the family therapy training program. If the core of the departmental faculty becomes disenchanted or threatened by the family therapy degree equivalent program because of high levels of student interest or for other reasons, students may feel triangulated between faculty representing the two professions. Thus, it is most important that departmental faculty acknowledge family therapy as a profession of equal status and importance with the parent profession if a Level-One program is to be successfully implemented.

An additional consideration arises if the Level-One program requires the coordination of core courses from several departments. It is helpful if close working relationships are established with the faculty of contributing departments. Frequently, faculty from other departments are more than willing to modify their courses so that they relate more directly to family therapy when their courses are components of the required family therapy curriculum.

Level Two: Family Therapy as a Professional Specialty

Level-Two training recognizes and defines family therapy as a subset of another mental health profession taught entirely within the structure of the degree program of that parent profession. Thus, a family therapy specialty is a program of limited scope and planned sequential study, complementing and adding to the core curriculum of the professional degree. Examples of Level-Two Professional Specialty programs occur within degree granting programs such as psychiatry, family medicine, psychology, counseling and guidance, clinical social work, and pastoral counseling. The key differences between Level-One and Level-Two programs are (a) the Level-One program is viewed as a degree or degree-equivalent program in family therapy while the Level-Two program is viewed as a professional specialty or concentration in family therapy supporting another professional degree program and (b) while both offer planned and sequential programs of study in family therapy, the Level-Two program is more limited in scope than the Level-One program.

Level-Two Curriculum. Level-Two curriculum for the family therapy professional specialty commonly includes a limited number of sequenced and planned courses identified as areas of study within Table 1. Within the areas of Marital and Family Systems and Therapy, fewer courses are offered and required than at Level-One. Individual Development courses usually are similar at both Levels-One and Two with respect to both the content and number of required courses, as these courses generally apply toward the departmental degree requirements as well as the MFT specialty requirements. Professional Studies at Level-Two differ from Level-One in that course content emphasizes individually oriented issues in psychotherapy, as well as socialization within the parent profession. Professional issues in family therapy are covered as a specific course component. Research as an area of study at Level-Two covers the broad spectrum of behavioral sciences research, including research in family therapy. Electives at Level-Two may provide additional coursework in family therapy or may be more closely related to the primary focus of the parent profession.

The Professional Specialty family therapy training sequence at Level-Two provides the trainee with the theoretical and clinical background to evaluate and treat, under the supervision of an experienced family therapy supervisor, a variety of marital and family problems. Trainees will be equipped to make appropriate referrals to a professional family therapist with educational and clinical training at Level-One when the family or couple is extremely resistive, exhibits intense systemic dysfunction, or does not respond to therapeutic interventions.

Level-Two Supervised Clinical Training. The Level-Two MFT Professional Specialization provides a supervised clinical practice that includes a limited number of clients presenting marital and/or family problems. This MFT clinical experience generally occurs within the framework of a general psychotherapy practicum or internship. An academically and clinically qualified family therapy supervisor should be responsible for the supervision of MFT cases in the clinical experience.

Level-One and Level-Two clinical training programs differ in that most Level-One programs offer their initial MFT clinical training block within a university operated family therapy clinical/training center (see Figure 1). The Level-Two program generally offers fewer opportunities to work with couples and families than a Level-One program.

Considerations. The strength of this model is that definitionally, the family therapy training occurs within the boundaries of a parent profession, thus minimizing the potential of a two-profession one-department conflict. The weakness of the Level-Two model is that it generally does not prepare students as completely in family therapy as they need or desire to attain their professional goals. Usually students from Level-Two programs require both additional coursework and clinical supervision prior to seeking Clinical Membership in the American Association for Marriage and Family Therapy.

Level-Three: Family Therapy Elective Study

Level-Three programs offer an *ad hoc* study of family therapy through offerings such as elective graduate courses, continuing education programs, and/or in-service training. A Level-Three program is designed to broaden the theoretical and conceptual base of therapists, preparing them to work in a limited role with couples and families. Thus, Level-Three training proposes limited objectives for therapists who will encounter occasional marriage and family related issues in their work with clients.

Curriculum. Curriculum at the Elective Level is offered on an *ad hoc* basis to students who seek to gain a basic understanding of the principles of family therapy to use in their work with clients. These courses are viewed as augmentation to individual and group oriented therapeutic training. The Elective Level (Level-Three) and Specialization Level (Level-Two) differ in that the Level-Three elective program is not a planned sequence of family therapy study and generally includes fewer courses than the Level-Two Family Therapy specialization. The Elective Level of family therapy training allows each student the latitude to select any, all, or none of the family therapy courses offered, depending on individual needs and interests.

The Elective Level of training generally includes an introduction to family therapy and Marital and Family Systems, perhaps combined in a single course. Level-Three training may offer coursework in areas related to parent education and family enrichment. Individual Development, as in Level-Two, is covered by the requirements of the core degree program. Professional Studies at Level-Three provides an overview of issues and trends in psychotherapy. The course is similar to the Level-Two Professional Studies course in that a specific focus on family therapy issues may be a single component of the course, if present at all. Finally, the Research component at Level-Three is designed to provide a broad overview of psychotherapy research. It may offer the individual student the opportunity to review family therapy research as a component of the course, but the review of family therapy research typically will not be a course requirement.

Supervised Clinical Practice. Clinical practice at the Family Therapy Elective Level of study does not include a planned sequence for skill development specifically in family therapy. Supervision is often provided by a qualified psychotherapist without specific training in family therapy. Clients that present family issues are responded to through the use of psychotherapeutic strategies taught within the context of the parent profession designed to promote individual change and growth. Level-Three training should prepare students with sufficient knowledge and skills to make appropriate referrals to Level-One and Two providers of family therapy when presenting issues are not resolved through interventions based on Level-Three training.

Considerations. Level-Three training is most appropriate to familiarize students with the applications of family therapy and to introduce them to the concept of working with couples and families to alleviate presenting problems in an individual. While Level-Three training may successfully introduce students to family therapy it has potential drawbacks: (a) it does not train therapists to work with families presenting complex systems problems; (b) it may confuse students by introducing only briefly the systems paradigm for change; and (c) it may encourage a few students to hold themselves out as family therapists when their training does not merit this. It is important that faculty and students at Level-Three be able to recognize the limitations of elective family therapy training. They should know when and when not to refer families to family therapists with more comprehensive professional training.

The major strengths of this level of training are: (a) it permits students in other mental health disciplines to be exposed to and gain some familiarity with family therapy; and (b) it may encourage students with strong interests in family therapy to pursue more in-depth post-graduate training in family therapy.

The potential problem of conflicting professional identities and dual professional affiliation that may occur at Level Two is rarely encountered within Level-Three programs, as family therapy is clearly defined as a sub-set of the parent profession.

PROFESSIONAL ISSUES RELATED TO IMPLEMENTATION

Perhaps the three most important questions that must be answered before a university implements a family therapy training program are (a) what are the basic goals and objectives of the training program, (b) how will family therapy relate to other psychotherapeutic paradigms currently taught, and (c) what level of the proposed training model will fit most congruently, considering the responses to a and b above? The answers to the aforementioned questions can only be obtained after an operational definition has been established for family therapy. It must be determined whether family therapy will be taught and treated as a profession or as a professional specialty within another discipline. Academicians must seek congruence between the program's goals and objectives, definition of family therapy, and the training model selected (Level-One, Two or Three). Departments that seek answers to the questions posed above prior to program implementation will experience a more harmonious transition into their family therapy training program and will expend considerably less effort initiating and maintaining the program.

Clarifying the Definition

Let us return to several basic questions. What is the relationship between family therapy and related professions? Is family therapy a sub-set of another profession or an independent profession in its own right? Models from set theory are useful to help conceptualize the potential relationships between family therapy and other mental health professions. In Figure 2a, family therapy is shown as a profession that is separate and distinct from other mental health care professions.

Such a definition of family therapy is congruent with family therapy degree programs implementing training at Level-One. In Figure 2b, family therapy is viewed as a partially overlapping set with another mental health discipline such as clinical or counseling psychology, clinical social work, pastoral counseling, professional counseling or psychiatry. This definition of family therapy also lends itself to Level-One training. Thus, Figures 2a and 2b illustrate the point-of-view that family therapy may be taught as a profession either alone or concurrently with one of the parent professions. Both Figures 2a and 2b represent valid models of family therapy for a Level-One training program. Such training programs may ultimately qualify for accreditation by the Commission on Accreditation for Marriage and Family Therapy Education.

All academic institutions, however, will not desire a Level-One family therapy training program. A set theory model for a program that seeks a Level-Two Professional Specialty family therapy training program is shown in Figure 2c. In this model, family therapy is clearly defined as a sub-set entirely within the boundaries of the parent profession. Such programs view family therapy as a professional specialty contributing to the body of knowledge of the parent profession.

The Level-Three training model is represented by Figure 2d. In this situation, the small sub-sets within the larger set represent courses in family therapy that are not organized in a planned, sequential fashion to offer a family therapy specialization. Rather, these family therapy courses are offered at the elective level to enhance interested students' knowledge of family therapy.

ISSUES OF PROFESSIONAL IDENTITY AND AFFILIATION

The relationship between two professional programs sharing equally within a single administrative unit is usually difficult. Wedding the two programs within an academic department requires considerable good-will and skill in diplomacy and negotiation. As is often the case, family therapy may be viewed as a new and immature profession more worthy of stepchild status than true brotherhood. Another issue is that family therapy is frequently very popular with students, who generate high levels of enthusiasm for instructors and courses in family therapy. If this enthusiasm is seen as drawing students away from the more traditional subject matter of the parent academic department, problems may arise.

Figure 2.
Relationship of Family Therapy to Other Mental Health Professions

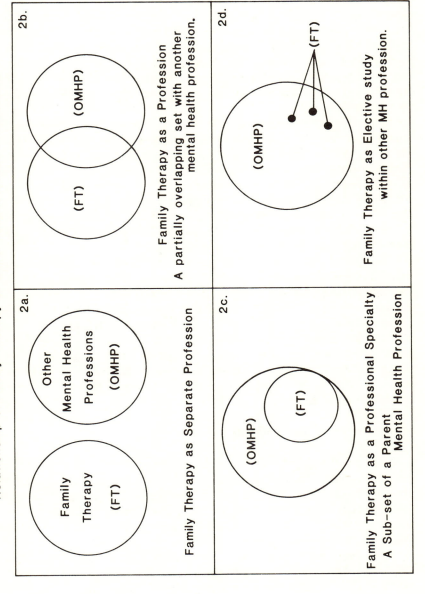

2a.

Family Therapy (FT)

Other Mental Health Professions (OMHP)

Family Therapy as Separate Profession

2b.

(FT)

(OMHP)

Family Therapy as a Profession
A partially overlapping set with another
mental health profession.

2c.

(OMHP)

(FT)

Family Therapy as a Professional Specialty
A Sub-set of a Parent
Mental Health Profession

2d.

(OMHP)

(FT)

Family Therapy as Elective study
within other MH profession.

Another significant issue in family therapy program integration is that of professional identification or allegiance for family therapy educators (Piercy and Hovestadt, 1980). The American Association for Marriage and Family Therapy (AAMFT) is recognized as the largest and most established professional organization for family therapists. When family therapy co-exists at a professional level within a parent department, the majority of faculty within that department may affiliate primarily with other professional associations. This situation may place family therapy faculty and students in an awkward position if they chose primary affilliation with AAMFT.

Academic representation is also an important issue. For example, should the family therapy educator represent him/herself within the department as a family therapist or as a member of the older parent profession? If the faculty member chooses to be identified as a family therapist, issues of loyalty and commitment to the parent profession may be raised by colleagues which may again place the family therapy faculty member in an uncomfortable position. Such seemingly insignificant points as those mentioned may result in ill-feelings among faculty and students if not detected early and resolved openly.

Piercy and Hovestadt (1980) point out that despite the difficulty of maintaining dual professional affiliations, it is often important for family therapy educators to make themselves an integral part of the professional support system of both AAMFT and the parent discipline. Such dual affiliation may be maintained through publications, participation in convention presentations, and serving in state and national leadership positions both within AAMFT and within the parent professional associations. Even dual professional affiliation, however, is not sufficient to guarantee harmony if clear goals and definitions for the family therapy training program are not established.

Professionalism and Political Reality

The three levels of training presented here offer various ways family therapy may be included in graduate education. The effects each of these training models will have on the development of a professional identity among program graduates and the political influence of family therapy in the marketplace will vary considerably and should be understood prior to implementation of any level of training.

The Level-One training model meets standards for accreditation by the American Association for Marriage and Family Therapy. Thus, this level of training develops a clear sense of professional identity as a family therapist among students in such programs. Additionally, this level of training produces graduates who serve as spokespersons for the profession of family therapy and are able to present family therapy as a unique and valuable profession to the public served.

The Level-Two and Level-Three training models tend to view family therapy as a component of another mental health care profession. Level-Two and Three programs promote the professional identity of the parent profession and view family therapy as one therapeutic modality among several possessed by graduates. Graduates of Level-Two and Three programs are more likely to emphasize their parent profession and may do little to increase the influence of the profession of family therapy to the consumer public. On the other hand, it should be remembered that family therapy training must begin somewhere, and that certain graduates of Level-Two and Three programs will develop a strong interest in family therapy and the systems paradigm and may choose to continue their family therapy education in post-graduate training institutes.

CONCLUSION

The primary and perhaps overriding issue pertaining to any level of integration of family therapy education is whether there is sufficient faculty support present to establish and maintain that program at the particular training level selected. Successful integration requires the support of an entire faculty. What seems clear is that before any concrete steps are made toward any level of implementation of family therapy education, departmental responses to the following question should be sought.

1. Is family therapy considered a profession or a sub-set of another mental health care profession?
2. Do the advantages of beginning a new program that may attract additional students outweigh the possible disadvantages?
3. What level of MFT training is desired?
4. Are sufficiently qualified faculty and physical resources available to support the program at the desired level?
5. Does a sufficient reservoir of faculty goodwill exist to resolve the issues that may arise from concurrently offering programs with intrapsychic and interpersonal/systemic philosophies.
6. Do mechanisms exist within the department to work through the inevitable conflicts that will arise?

Once these questions are addressed the difficult task of implementing the family therapy training program at the desired level may begin. Like any process, there will be an element of trial-and-error involved. However, potential problems may be reduced through consideration of the training model and recommendations presented here.

REFERENCES

Broderick, C.B. (1981). Personal Communication referenced in Gurman, A.S. and Kniskern, D.P. (Eds.), *Handbook of family therapy,* New York: Brunner/Mazel.

Broderick, C.B. and Schrader, S.S. (1981). The history of professional marriage and family therapy. In A.S. Gurman, and D.P. Kniskern, (Eds.), *Handbook of family therapy,* New York: Brunner/Mazel.

Burr, W.R. and Leigh, G.K. (1983). Famology: A new discipline. *Journal of Marriage and the Family, 45,* 467-480.

Cooper, J. and Charnofsky, S. (1983). Curricula and program development in marriage and family counseling: Process and content. In B.F. Okun and S.T. Gladding (Eds.), *Issues in training marriage and family therapists* (pp. 5-16). Ann Arbor, MI: ERIC/CAPS.

Gurman, A.S. and Kniskern, D.P. (Eds.), (1981). *Handbook of family therapy,* New York: Brunner/Mazel.

Hovestadt, A., Fenell, D. and Piercy, F. (1983). Integrating marriage and family therapy within counselor education: A three-level model. In B. Okun and S. Gladding (Eds.), *Issues in training marriage and family therapists* (p. 31-42). Ann Arbor, MI: ERIC/CAPS.

Johnson, A.S. III. (1984). AAMFT profile: Growth and opportunity, *Family Therapy News.* May-June, 20.

Liddle, H. and Halpin, R. (1978). Family therapy training and supervision: A comparative review. *Journal of Marriage and Family Counseling, 4,* 77-98.

Marriage and Family Therapy: Manual on Accreditation (1981). Washington, D.C.: American Association for Marriage and Family Therapy, Commission on Accreditation for Marriage and Family Therapy Education.

Olson, D.H., Russell, C.S., and Sprenkle, D.H. (1980). Marital and family therapy: A decade review. *Journal of Marriage and the Family, 42,* 973-994.

Piercy, F. and Hovestadt, A. (1980). Marriage and Family therapy within counselor education. *Counselor Education and Supervision, 20* (1), 68-74.

Piercy, F., Hovestadt, A., Fenell, D., Franklin, E., and McKeon, D. (1982). A comprehensive training model for family therapists serving rural populations. *Family Therapy, 9* (3), 239-249.

Thomas, M. (1983). A comparison of CACREP and AAMFT requirements for accreditation. In B. Okun and S. Gladding (Eds.), *Issues in training marriage and family therapists,* (pp. 17-27). Ann Arbor, MI: ERIC/CAPS.

An Insider's Comparison
of a Major Family Therapy
Doctoral Program and a Leading Nondegree
Family Therapy Training Center

Philip M. Sutton

ABSTRACT. This paper presents the author's experience of family therapy training in the doctoral program in Marriage and Family Therapy at Purdue University and in the Post-Doctoral Clinical Psychology Internship and Weekly Extern programs at the Philadelphia Child Guidance Clinic. The author describes each of the programs, compares their major features, and suggests general considerations for choosing either a doctoral program or a nondegree training center in order to learn family therapy.

In the present paper, I will describe and compare my recent experiences of family therapy training in the Marriage and Family Therapy Doctoral Program at Purdue University and in the Post-Doctoral Clinical Psychology Internship at the Philadelphia Child Guidance Clinic (PCGC). I conducted my doctoral work at Purdue from August, 1980 until August, 1983; and I served the internship at PCGC from September, 1983 until August, 1984. While the internship is more accurately described as a fellowship, I refer to the PCGC clinical psychology training program as an internship because that is the name by which it is known at PCGC. (At PCGC, physicians at all levels of training—medical student, intern, and pediatric or psychiatric resident—are called 'fellows', while psychologists in the post-doctoral training program are called 'interns'.) I also will describe my observations of another training program at PCGC, the Weekly Extern Program based on my contacts with some of the Extern faculty and externs. The PCGC Weekly Extern Program is more typical of the training available in nondegree family therapy training centers across the country than is the Clinical Psychology Internship.

I write this paper in the first person, as a professional with an "insider's" perspective regarding family therapy training at both a nationally prominent doctoral program and a leading training center of fam-

Philip M. Sutton, Ph.D., is a Psychologist and Family Therapist at the Family Learning Center, 1513 Miami Street, South Bend, IN 46617.

41

ily therapy. I have chosen to label PCGC as 'nondegree' even though PCGC cosponsors a program with the University of Pennsylvania Graduate School of Education (of which I was not a part) which leads to a master's degree in psychological services from the University of Pennsylvania and a certificate of training in family therapy from PCGC. (PCGC staff teach theory courses in family therapy and supervise the students in one of the Weekly Extern groups.) While my experience at PCGC and Purdue may not be generalizable to all family therapy doctoral programs and training centers, my observations and experiences raise questions that may be useful for mental health professionals who are interested in family therapy training across a variety of training contexts.

DESCRIPTIONS OF THE PROGRAMS

Marriage and Family Therapy Program at Purdue University

The Marriage and Family Therapy Program at Purdue University (MFT-PU) is housed in the Department of Child Development and Family Studies, an interdisciplinary department which combines graduate programs in Child Development, Family Studies, Early Childhood Education, Parent and Family Life Education, and Marriage and Family Therapy. The MFT-PU Program educates master's trained professionals from a variety of disciplines (e.g., clinical, counseling, and school psychology; social work; pastoral counseling; psychiatric nursing; family studies; etc.) as family therapists using a scientist/practitioner model which stresses the integration of research, theory, and practice (Olson, 1976).

The family therapy core curriculum includes four courses in family therapy theory which cover general systems theory and the major schools of family therapy (see Gurman and Kniskern, 1981a, for a review of the major schools), a survey course on family therapy outcome research, and elective specialized courses including marriage and family enrichment, sex therapy, divorce therapy, premarital therapy, and family therapy with substance abusers. MFT-PU students are required to take clinical practica for two out of every three semesters while in residence—the curriculum is designed to last at least three years—and a practicum in family therapy supervision. Other training experiences include a community field placement and an opportunity to lead a therapy or enrichment group. A key facet of the doctoral preliminary examination is the MFT Specialization Examination which involves writing an integrative paper describing the theory one uses to practice family therapy and presenting the paper to MFT-PU faculty and students along with edited videotapes of one's own family therapy which illustrates one's theory and practice.

MFT-PU students also take a curriculum of general theory and research courses including survey courses in child development, family studies, and general theory construction, and courses in statistics and research design. These courses, plus requirements to write scholarly papers in various classes and elective opportunities to participate in research projects, provide the background for designing and implementing one's doctoral dissertation research.

Philadelphia Child Guidance Clinic

PCGC is a multi-disciplinary facility organized to provide service and training and to conduct research devoted to caring for the mental health needs of children and their families. PCGC is affiliated with the Children's Hospital of the University of Pennsylvania's School of Medicine. PCGC staffs and houses the Children Hospital's psychiatric inpatient unit which provides short-term (30 day maximum) hospitalization. PCGC is also a community mental health center for Philadelphia County, Pennsylvania, and provides both inpatient and outpatient services to persons living in the PCGC catchment area of West and Southwest Philadelphia. In addition, PCGC operates the Family Therapy Training Center, providing family therapy training and continuing education programs in a variety of formats to mental health professionals. Both the Clinical Psychology Internship and the Weekly Extern Program are conducted by the Family Therapy Training Center.

Clinical Psychology Internship. The Clinical Psychology Internship at PCGC is a twelve month program specializing in child psychology and family therapy. The internship provides a post-doctoral or second, specialized internship experience for trainees who have already completed a predoctoral, general psychology internship. Interns, whose backgrounds could be clinical, counseling, or school psychology (my Master's work was in clinical psychology) focus on learning how to use psychological assessments of children as systemic intervention (Ziffer, 1984) and how to do structural family therapy.

Approximately half of the work week is spent delivering therapeutic services and receiving supervision on the therapy. Another fifth of the time is devoted to performing psychological assessments of children, staffing completed test batteries, and receiving supervision on the sessions in which we communicated the results of the assessments to the children, their families, and their PCGC therapists. The remainder of the week is spent in more specialized service or training opportunities.

The other interns and I participated in weekly seminars and received supervision of our intake work as members of the team which assesses crisis referrals to PCGC's inpatient units. We also received weekly seminar supervision of our duties as PCGC liasons and/or consultants to Philadelphia area public schools. There are regular opportunities to attend presentations by senior staff clinicians who describe the results of their research and clinical work on the family therapy treatment of clients with various presenting problems: anorexia nervosa, asthma, bulimia, sickle cell anemia, deafness, diabetes, divorce-related concerns, gastrointestinal problems, etc. The work with such a wide variety of problems is facilitated by PCGC's being affiliated with and housed adjacent to the Children's Hospital of the University of Pennsylvania which provides many referrals and requests for consultations. Although past intern groups have provided psychological consultations to the Hospital, my group did not have the opportunity to do so.

Available is an extensive collection of both edited and unedited videotapes of both prominent (e.g., Minuchin, Montalvo, Fishman, etc.) and relatively unknown therapists treating diverse forms of families with a wide variety of presenting problems. We used these videotapes for both planned and unplanned (i.e., no show or cancelled sessions) training opportunities. Because PCGC is a county mental health center, interns also participate with all other clinicians in weekly case review conferences led by PCGC psychiatrists in order to meet county and state requirements for case management.

Weekly Extern Program. The weekly extern program is the primary training program of the Family Therapy Training Center at PCGC. These externs meet for one full day per week from October through May for clinical work and supervision and for an entire day each month for didactic presentations. Externs are organized around teams of two senior staff supervisors and eight extern trainees. Externs are selected from applicants from all of the many professions who provide therapeutic services. Externs usually maintain full-time employment while participating in the weekly clinical and monthly didactic training.

Extern days involve reviewing videotapes of the previous week's sessions in the morning and experiencing live supervision of four consecutive hourly therapy sessions by each supervisor in the afternoon. Externs have the opportunity to experience live supervision of their own case for one hour and of other extern's cases for three hours. Extern groups also have access to the videotape library. When extern groups were begun at PCGC in 1975, the supervisors included many therapists who were or became nationally prominent (e.g., Salvador Minuchin and Jay Haley).

During the 1983-84 extern year, there were six different extern groups, most of which were not led by nationally prominent clinicians. Although current extern groups do not have the contact with the prominent PCGC clinicians that former extern groups once had, current extern groups still appear to have highly skilled and experienced clinicians as their supervisors. An informal consensus of opinion among PCGC staff suggests that the less well-known staff often prove to be more approachable and easier to learn from than many of the more well-known staff members of the past. PCGC also conducts other extern groups, including ones that meet monthly and for three consecutive weeks during the summer at PCGC and ones that meet at various time intervals in other cities.

COMPARISONS OF THE MFT-PU
AND PCGC PROGRAMS

Family Therapy Training

The MFT-PU Program conducts family therapy training using a live supervision model supplemented with videotape and case report supervision. The training practica are usually six to seven hours long and allow for as many as three consecutive sessions in three different time slots. Trainees typically are supervised by either the faculty supervisor or an advanced graduate student with prior experience and training in supervision. Occasionally, the supervisor is a ''supervisor-in-training'' from the practicum in supervision (Constantine, Piercy, & Sprenkle, 1984). Practicum trainees who are not seeing clients at a given time slot typically follow a particular case, forming a therapeutic and/or supervisory team as negotiated by the designated supervisor and therapist. The function of this team is similar to that described by Coppersmith (1980). Time is allotted to discuss the case and to process the session both before and after the live supervision. In addition to case management issues, a frequent focus of supervision is the consideration and facilitation of therapists' integration of their professed theoretical orientation with their clinical practice. In addition to practicum supervision, students also receive one hour per week of one-to-one supervision from the practicum supervisor. Since MFT-PU practica typically require caseloads of only five cases per week, supervision time per case is maximized.

The PCGC extern and clinical psychology intern programs also are conducted using a live supervision format with supplemental videotape supervision. In the internship, interns had a three hour time block in which two cases were supervised live and processed similar to the MFT-PU practicum. Interns who were not doing therapy in the session observed with the supervisor, but the experience provided more observational learning than an opportunity to serve as a therapeutic team. Interns also received two hours of individual supervision per week from another supervisor who gave the primary supervision of the interns' caseload of twelve cases per week. One of these hours was typically spent in live supervision and the other hour in case report or videotape supervision. The higher caseload in the internship allowed for little or no supervision of many cases but also provided a depth of experience that the lighter MFT-PU caseloads could not.

The format of the family therapy training in the PCGC extern program has already been described above. Externs receive supervision on only one case per week, although they are able to observe the cases of three other therapists. The supervision is confined to the one hour allotted to the case and to videotape observation and discussion the following week. Such a tight schedule appeared to leave little time for processing the case and exploring theoretical or general clinical issues raised by a given case. The limited caseload also left the externs at risk for receiving no direct supervision if their only client failed to come for the session. The major advantage of the extern program was that it provided mental health professionals who were already working the opportunity to receive intensive direct and observational training in family therapy while continuing to work. The support provided by the other members of the extern group was also a substantial aid to and benefit of the extern training format.

Theoretical Focus

The MFT-PU program espouses an overall family systems and orientation in training, but only one of the four full-time faculty supervise with a clearly focused theoretical orientation (i.e., structural/strategic). The program encourages therapists to explore, differentiate, and integrate the variety of historical and current theoretical orientations, and to learn to practice consistent with the orientation which one chooses. Although some students enter the program with extensive training in one of the family therapy orientations and continue to affirm that orientation, other and perhaps most students enter without having adopted an orientation and are challenged to adopt one. I have observed that students and faculty are very influenced by the latest trends in family therapy theory and training methods that appear in the literature.

For example, the students preceding my class appeared to have concentrated on practicing structural family therapy and Milan-team strategic therapy, while my class and other classes appear to have concentrated on Haley or MRI strategic approaches, as well as functional family therapy (see Gurman & Kniskern, 1981a, for a description of the approaches). The interests of the students and the flexibility and interests of the faculty appear to allow for and to foster different therapeutic orientations and training methods.

Both the PCGC intern and extern programs are organized to teach structural family therapy (Minuchin, 1974; Minuchin & Fishman, 1981). This orientation or "school" of family therapy was developed extensively and popularized primarily at PCGC. Although all of the supervisors

with whom I had contact claimed to be ''eclectic'' regarding the use of interventions, each conceptualized cases structurally and espoused therapeutic strategies and interventions that have been widely associated with
structural family therapy. Treatment interventions were recommended
and evaluated according to how well the interventions would meet (or had
met) the mediating and ultimate (Gurman & Kniskern, 1981b) treatment
goals from a structural perspective.

PCGC staff rarely mentioned ''structural family therapy'' by name;
rather, the staff taught ''family therapy,'' sometimes referring to what
Sal (Minuchin) had said or would do. I never heard PCGC staff either
publically or privately trying to integrate or accommodate the structural
approach with other approaches to family therapy, which was a big
change from my experience at MFT-PU. I did, however, perceive a willingness to consider whether and how interventions associated with other
family therapy and non-family therapy orientations could be used to effect
structural outcomes. PCGC staff clearly use non-structural interventions,
particularly strategic techniques and, where appropriate, such non-family
therapy techniques as hospitalization, medicine, psychological testing,
peer groups, biofeedback, and hypnosis (Ziffer, 1984). But the staff
follow a guideline that practical and theoretical eclecticism may be prac-
tised more successfully after trainees have mastered a coherent practical
and conceptual approach to family therapy.

Professionalization

The MFT-PU program is accredited by the American Association for
Marriage and Family Therapy (AAMFT) to educate doctoral trained
marriage and family therapists. As described above, the MFT-PU program draws students from a variety of professional disciplines and
teaches the theory, research, and practice of family therapy. But the program also effects membership in a new profession (i.e., family therapy)
and fosters the socialization of a new professional identity (i.e., family
therapist). Although AAMFT has acknowledged the tension between promoting a new profession of family therapists and serving the needs of
mental health professionals who do family therapy but whose initial or
primary identification is with one of the ''traditional four professions''
(Williamson, 1979, 1980), the MFT-PU program is designed to train
family therapists, not psychologists, social workers, counselors, etc., to
do family therapy. I did not find much help while in the MFT-PU program in resolving the tension I felt in trying to integrate my orientation
and skills as a family therapist with my master's level training in clinical
psychology. In order to maintain better my identity as a psychologist, I
applied for admission into the clinical psychology internship at PCGC.

In the clinical psychology internship at PCGC, interns learn how to practice as psychologists from a structural family therapy perspective. We were taught to be "family psychologists," to use the process and outcomes of psychological evaluations as interventions into the systems of the individual being assessed, the family, and the broader social context including school, employment, etc. We also were taught to be "family therapists" along with trainees from psychiatry, social work, and psychiatric nursing. Trainees from each professional discipline were taught how to do structural family therapy, but also how to use the knowledge and skills that are specific to their profession to achieve structural goals. For example, psychiatric fellows are taught how to use medication and hospitalization to help families achieve the desired structural changes. This approach to training different mental health professionals to do structural family therapy has evolved and is reinforced by the medical model under which PCGC must operate as a community mental health center and in its affiliation with the Children's Hospital of the University of Pennsylvania's School of Medicine.

The PCGC extern program attempts to train mental health professionals to do family therapy. I perceived no direct efforts by PCGC extern faculty either to promote a new profession or professional identity as a family therapist, or to help externs use the adjunctive therapies of their professions-of-origin (e.g., medicine, psychological testing, etc.) in a systematic way. However, externs were encouraged to make referrals to PCGC staff if adjunctive therapeutic interventions were judged desirable. Such referrals would lead to collaboration with PCGC professionals who in the context of their professional roles would model how to use the specialized skills of a nurse, psychiatrist, psychologist, or social worker with a structural family therapy orientation.

SUGGESTED CRITERIA FOR DECIDING WHERE TO RECEIVE FAMILY THERAPY TRAINING

Part-Time vs. Full-Time Availability for Training

Weekly, monthly, or week long intensive extern programs at training centers such as PCGC seem ideal to me for professionals who want to learn to do family therapy and who choose (or have) to remain employed full-time. I would discourage professionals from choosing a graduate program, especially a doctoral program, unless they are prepared to make it a primary time commitment, especially for the pre-dissertation phase of the program. Valuable extracurricular contacts with supervisors and fellow students are more difficult to maintain for students not in full-time residence.

Desired Professional Identity and Kind of Degree

One's current profession and career goals will influence whether one should choose an academic setting or a clinical training center in order to learn family therapy. For example, individuals wanting the most thorough academic education in family therapy probably will find it in a university graduate program in family therapy. Similarly, professionals who desire a change in career (e.g., from school psychology to family therapy) or want to acquire a degree which allows a wider range of job opportunities (e.g., augmenting a master's degree in counseling, psychology, or social work, or a bachelor's degree in nursing or any of the social or behavioral sciences) should consider earning a degree from an academic training program in family therapy. There are a growing number of both master's and doctoral degree granting programs in family therapy around the country, many of which are accredited by AAMFT.[1] Professionals from the traditional mental health fields of psychiatry, clinical/counseling psychology, social work, or psychiatric nursing who do *not* want to adopt the professional identity of "family therapist" or who do not want to teach family therapy in an academic setting, may wish to seek nondegree training instead.

Type of Training Available

I believe that live supervision is the supervisory mode of choice for beginning family therapists. I also believe that the more experience professionals have in working with individuals, couples, and families from a family systems framework, the more useful they will find trying to integrate family systems concepts with their practice. The value of a training setting being theoretically heterogeneous or homogeneous will vary according to the personality, flexibility, and previous experience of the trainee, and the skill of the supervisor/trainer. In general, (having experienced training first in a theoretically heterogeneous setting and then in a theoretically more homogeneous setting) I believe that it is easier for beginners to learn family therapy first in a setting which teaches one specific approach.

Regardless of whether the training setting is degree or nondegree granting, I would encourage *new* family therapists to choose the theoretically more homogenous setting which affords the greater measure of live supervision and the larger caseloads. For more experienced therapists, a theoretically more diverse approach to training and supervision may be appropriate. Also, more experienced therapists not wishing to earn another degree or professionals who work in places where few opportunities exist for family therapy training, might find appropriate training in small group or individual supervision sessions in a training center, institute, or private practice setting. Many supervisors of family therapy are accredited by AAMFT.[1]

CONCLUSION

I value highly my doctoral training in the Marriage and Family Therapy Program at Purdue University because of the depth and breadth of education in family therapy theories and practices, the opportunities to teach, supervise, and do research, and the faculty and their quality supervision which helped me begin my career as a family therapist. I also value my intern year at the Philadelphia Child Guidance Clinic where the more extensive clinical experience, the quality of supervision, and the more theoretically focused orientation helped me to develop more competency and confidence as a family therapist. My year at PCGC has also enabled me to integrate better my training and identity as a psychologist with my MFT-PU training and professionalization as a family therapist. Also, I enjoy having worked and trained where Salvador Minuchin, a patriarch of family therapy, did such memorable work and training—I think many of the PCGC trainees chose PCGC for similar reasons. Finally, I value the supervision and training done at my present place of employment, a private practice agency. I am pleased that I have been able to receive from each setting the training which I desired and expected.

My closing comment to professionals in the process of choosing a setting in which to receive training in family therapy is: Decide what your personal and professional expectations and constraints are, and then "shop around." Compare the programs offered by universities, agencies, training centers, institutes, and/or private supervisors and choose the setting which best meets your personal and professional expectations, constraints, and preferences.

REFERENCES

Constantine, J., Piercy, F., & Sprenkle, D. (1984). Live supervision of supervision in family therapy. *Journal of Marital and Family Therapy, 10,* 95-97.
Coopersmith, E. (1980). Expanding uses of the telephone in family therapy. *Family Process, 19,* 411-417.
Gurman, A., & Kniskern, D. (Eds.). (1981). *Handbook of family therapy.* New York: Brunner/Mazel. (a)
Gurman, A., & Kniskern, D. (1981). Family therapy outcome research: Knowns and unknowns.

[1]A list of universities and training centers with AAMFT-accredited programs in marriage and family therapy is included at the end of this volume. A list of AAMFT-approved supervisors in your area can be obtained by writing: AAMFT, 1717 K Street NW # 407, Washington, D.C. 20006.

In A. Gurman & D. Kniskern (Eds.), *Handbook of family therapy* (pp. 742-775). New York: Brunner/Mazel. (b)

Minuchin, S. (1974). *Families and family therapy.* Cambridge: Harvard University Press.

Minuchin, S., & Fishman, C. (1981). *Family therapy techniques.* Cambridge: Harvard University Press.

Olson, D. (1976). Bridging research, theory, and application: The triple threat in science. In D. Olson (Ed.), *Treating relationships* (pp. 565-579). Lake Mills, IA: Graphic.

Williamson, D. (1979). Board or bored? [Opinion from the president.] *Family Therapy News.* September, 2, 7.

Williamson, D. (1980). Closing remarks [From the president]. *Family Therapy News,* November, 2, 4, 6, 9.

Ziffer, R. (1984). *Adjunctive techniques in family therapy.* Orlando, FL: Grune and Stratton.

Rethinking Family Therapy Education and Supervision: A Feminist Model

Dorothy Wheeler
Judith Myers Avis
Lorie A. Miller
Sita Chaney

ABSTRACT. Feminism challenges the way in which family therapy is currently conceptualized and practiced as well as the way in which therapists are trained and supervised. This article proposes a model which delineates perceptual, conceptual, and executive skills in a feminist approach to family therapy. These skills are discussed in relation to three phases of therapy: a) developing and maintaining a working alliance between the family and the therapist, b) defining the problem, and c) facilitating change. Issues related to teaching these skills in both the classroom and supervision are examined.

Although feminist family therapy has been discussed in the literature since 1976 (Hare-Mustin, 1978, 1979; Seidler-Feller, 1976), there has been no clearly defined framework for identifying the specific skills characteristic of such therapy or for the training of therapists. This article addresses this gap by presenting a model of feminist family therapy which includes skills and appropriate training methodologies.

Feminism is not a set of techniques or conclusions but rather a lens through which one views and understands realities. Feminism, according to Wheeler (1983), is "a process that begins with the recognition of the inferior status of women, proceeds to an analysis of the specific forms and causes of that inequality, makes recommendations for strategies of

Author's names are listed in random order and reflect equal contribution to this collaborative paper.

Dorothy Wheeler, M.S., Judith Myers Avis, M.S.W., and Sita Chaney, M.S. are doctoral students in the Family Therapy Doctoral Program, Department of Child Development and Family Studies, Purdue University, West Lafayette, IN 47907. In addition, Judith Myers Avis is an Assistant Professor of Social Work (on leave), St. Thomas University, Fredericton, New Brunswick, Canada E3B 5G3.

Lorie A. Miller, B.S.W., is Director of Counseling, Planned Parenthood, Lafayette, Indiana and Research Consultant for the Labor Studies Project, Department of Child Development and Family Studies, Purdue University, West Lafayette, Indiana.

53

change, and eventually leads to a recognition and validation of women's realities, women's interpretations, and women's contributions'' (p. 1). As a method of analysis, feminism implies an active process as opposed to a static set of conclusions. Hartsock (1975) defines feminism as a ''method of approaching life and politics, a way of asking questions and searching for answers'' (p. 68).

FEMINIST CRITIQUES OF FAMILY THERAPY

Systems theory, the foundation upon which much of family therapy is built, has been criticized by feminists for its abstract, ahistorical, and apolitical assumptions (James & McIntyre, 1983). With its emphasis on circular causality, systems theory virtually has ignored gender inequality within the family. Family dysfunctions typically are assumed to be a result of interpersonal dynamics, rather than a reflection of larger social influences that encourage inequality on the basis of sex. By ignoring social forces, family therapists inadvertently participate in maintaining their negative consequences (James & McIntyre, 1983).

Family systems theory de-emphasizes the origins of family problems, contending that current and ongoing interaction is more important (Hoffman, 1981). Feminists, however, adopt a more linear model, one which views women's inferior position as having historical origins which continue to be reinforced in the family (Thorne & Yalom, 1982). When one ignores history, it is easy to assume mistakenly that women and men have equal impact on their surroundings.

Because family systems theory does not incorporate the history of gender inequality, women are considered by many family therapists to be as responsible as men in maintaining dysfunctional sequences. However, because men and women do not occupy equal positions of power in society, they cannot affect systems equally as the notion of circular causality seems to imply (Miller, 1983). To adhere to systems theory's circular view of causality is, at least in part, to blame the victim—in this case, women.

In addition to systems theory, other aspects of family therapy have been criticized. Jacobson (1983) argues that family therapists are not sensitive to power differences within the family which favor men. If treatment proceeds with the expectation that *each* partner change equally, then pretreatment inequities remain intact. Because families rarely define their concerns in terms of power imbalances caused by socialization, Jacobson (1983) suggests that the therapist has an ethical responsibility, regardless of presenting problem, to attempt to redistribute power.

Gurman and Klein (1984) suggest that much of family therapy operates within a system laden with gender bias which disadvantages women. The problem results because family therapists assert an "objective and data-based neutrality" (p. 185) and do not adopt a more critical examination of the values which they are implementing. Behavioral marital therapy (BMT), they argue, has a tendency to label behavior as "positive" or "negative." A "good" relationship or one that is positively valued within the BMT frame is one in which accommodation, personal sacrifice, and lack of conflict are the norm. When a wife who was formerly passive and non-assertive begins to demonstrate autonomy there is often an increase in marital conflict. This behavior cannot be seen as healthy because it is viewed systemically and labeled as negative. The value of this behavior to the individual is lost in a normative family framework insensitive to individual needs (Gurman & Klein, 1984).

Avis (in press), Gurman and Klein (1984), Hare-Mustin (1978), and others have criticized family therapy for emphasizing the importance of changing performance within roles rather than changing the roles themselves. Avis, for example, challenges Functional Family Therapy for its unequivocal support and legitimization of functions (i.e., the tendency of different family members to seek interpersonal closeness or distance). She asserts that these functions are not, in fact, idiosyncratic or personally chosen by family members. Rather they are correlated with traditionally prescribed gender role behavior, with closeness or merging functions (e.g., involvement with children) fulfilled primarily by women and distancing functions (e.g., time away from family) by men. Functional Family Therapy, Avis argues, actually perpetuates and encourages such sex role behavior.

The use of hierarchy in family therapy also has been criticized. Hare-Mustin (1978), in describing a feminist approach to family therapy, pays special attention to the structure of the relationship between the family and the therapist. She suggests the use of a therapist-family contract to minimize the therapeutic hierarchy, to set limits on the therapist's authority, and to provide the opportunity for all family members, but especially women, to negotiate individual and system needs. While Hare-Mustin's suggestions are important first steps in remedying sexism in family therapy, there appears to be a compelling need to develop a family therapy model with specific procedures sensitive to feminist issues.

FEMINIST FAMILY THERAPY: AN ALTERNATIVE

A feminist approach to family therapy incorporates many aspects of family systems thinking: a) an emphasis on social context as a prime determinant of behavior, b) the use of reframing and relabeling to shift the conceptual or emotional perspective on a situation, c) modeling, and d) an emphasis on action and behavioral change (Libow, Raskin, & Caust,

1982). A feminist approach also is similar to a non-sexist approach to family therapy in its commitment to facilitating equality in personal power between women and men, and in supporting clients' rights to design their lives outside of culturally prescribed sex roles (Rice & Rice, 1977).

What sets a feminist approach to family therapy apart from both traditional and nonsexist approaches, however, is its commitment to recognizing the *unique* problems women face as a result of their socialization, and a commitment to change that will benefit women (Gilbert, 1980). Additionally, most feminist perspectives on therapy emphasize the sharing of power in the therapeutic relationship rather than the usual therapist-client hierarchy. Moreover, feminist family therapy demands a more political, institutional, and gender-sensitive viewpoint which confronts familial and societal barriers so that women can exercise their individual choices and participate as equals with men. Perhaps as importantly, a feminist approach to family therapy must support and validate women's work both within and outside the family (Rowbotham, 1973). Feminist family therapy is distinguished from others forms of feminist therapy by its particular focus on changing family structure and its involvement of the family system in this process.

While men also have been victims of a sexist culture and its rigid patterns of socialization, it is still men who hold the balance of power and receive a disproportionate share of social rewards and privileges. A feminist approach is concerned with correcting this imbalance as it occurs within the family. The overall goal of integrating feminist ideas into family therapy is, therefore, to change the institution of the family so that those women and men who choose to participate in family life can do so cooperatively as equal and intimate partners. This formidable goal requires distinct ways of intervening, as well as a redefinition of healthy family functioning.

Alternative View of Healthy Family Functioning

Family Life Cycle: The family life cycle usually is discussed in terms of stereotypic roles for men and women. An integration of feminist ideas can broaden our thinking about family health and desirable therapeutic outcome to include and validate such options as a) remaining single and establishing intimacy from within a network of friendships; b) choosing a marriage without children; c) choosing to be a single parent; d) choosing divorce as a mature and responsible decision; e) choosing homosexual or heterosexual cohabitation with or without children; and f) generally questioning traditional ideas regarding gender-appropriate behaviors from within the family. Healthy outcome, in other words, can be broadened to include one's ability to withstand pressures to conform to stereotypic ideas about how families should be.

Equalization of Resources and Responsibility. In the traditional family, the wife has been expected to subordinate her interests to those of her family, while the husband has been expected to maximize his individuality and autonomy (Kolbenschlag, 1980). A feminist alternative would support *each* family member maximizing his/her individuality and autonomy, while at the same time sharing more or less equally in an accommodation or subordination of individual needs.

Roles. It is important to examine both the relationship between roles and gender and the processes by which roles are allocated. From a feminist perspective, a healthy family is one in which males and females have a wide range of roles available to them, and the allocation of roles by gender is minimal. In addition, roles should be decided on the basis of personal choice and interpersonal negotiation rather than as a result of sex role prescriptions (Klein, 1976).

Hierarchy and Health. Feminist theory suggests that hierarchical structures within (and outside) the family often restrict women (Thorne and Yalom, 1982). Haley (1976) argues that organization and hierarchy are one and the same and symptoms result when the hierarchy is confused or unclear.

Appropriate differences, separation, and generational boundaries can (and should) exist between individuals and subsystems within the family. However, Haley's emphasis on the inevitability of working out primary and secondary status positions determines a view of behavior and relationships as adversarial, competitive, and unstable. A healthy system, from a feminist perspective, would minimize same-generation hierarchical arrangements (particularly those based on gender), as well as power struggles that result from such arrangements.

Separating the Personal, Interpersonal, and Social. A healthy family, from a feminist perspective, is one in which the members understand the political and social influences on their personal or interpersonal lives. This often results in behaviors initially defined as personal inadequacies being reinterpreted as socially prescribed. Women and girls need to be helped to examine what it is they have been taught about being female in comparison to their actual competencies, interests, and needs. Men and boys need to examine what they have been taught about women. Additionally, both sexes can re-examine their socialized learnings regarding commitment, caretaking, and intimacy.

Individual vs. System Well-Being. Individual well-being and family well-being are equally important in feminist family therapy. Consequently when individual and family needs conflict, the family should not necessarily be supported at the expense of the individual. For example, if a woman returns to school or work this may threaten family stability. The feminist family therapist would support such a shift in structure and distribution of functions.

A MODEL OF FEMINIST FAMILY THERAPY

Tomm and Wright (1979) have developed a useful framework for delineating perceptual, conceptual, and executive family therapy skills. This framework will be used to present the requisite skills for a model of feminist family therapy. They refer to *perceptual/conceptual skills* as those "taking place in the mind of the therapist" (p. 228), with perception referring to "the therapist's ability to make pertinent and accurate observations" and conception being "the process of attributing meaning to observations or of applying previous learning to the specific therapeutic situation" (p. 229). Taken together, these comprise the therapist's thinking skills, and are so integrally interrelated that they are difficult to separate in practice. *Executive skills,* on the other hand, refer to the action or response of the therapist and include both the therapist's internal emotional reactions and overt therapeutic actions.

Because of the close relationship between thinking and acting, executive skills are dependent on an appropriate perceptual/conceptual base. Thus, although perceptual/conceptual and executive skills can be identified and discussed separately, in practice they form an integral whole, with the former providing a necessary foundation for the latter.

The present model of feminist family therapy presupposes that therapists either have, or are acquiring, basic family therapy competencies and does not detail all the skills in thinking and intervening necessary for effective work with families. Rather, this feminist model is intended to complement existing models of therapy and to elaborate those skills which are particularly feminist in their intent and focus. Since this is a first attempt to articulate such a feminist model, it is not intended to be exhaustive or definitive but rather to identify a variety of ways in which feminist ideology and goals can be integrated into family therapy practice. This model was developed from the authors' integration of feminist principles into their teaching, supervision, and therapy with families.

Perceptual/Conceptual Skills

A feminist conceptualization of the family provides the therapist with an expanded lens through which to observe and understand family relationships. The change in perception which results from such a conceptualization is analogous to that which occurs when a therapist shifts from a linear to a system/interactional paradigm. Such a shift changes the focus of therapeutic attention, the meaning the therapist attaches to observed behavior, the conceptualization of change, the intervention strategies selected from the purely interpersonal to the political.

In using a systemic lens, for example, the therapist views the behaviors of a nagging wife and withdrawing husband, not as isolated personality traits, but in the context of their relationship system. If the therapist then adds a feminist lens, s/he will begin to see "nagging" as a behavior of powerlessness and "withdrawing" as an exercise of power (Feldman, 1982). This view will influence the therapeutic goals sought and the interventions selected.

Interventions thus grow out of the way in which the therapist thinks about the family. As a result, feminist-informed skills cannot be taught simply through supervision, modeling, or microskill practice (Ivey, 1971). They can only be taught in conjunction with a thorough re-thinking and re-conceptualization of the relations between men and women both in society and in the family. These shifts in thinking provide the foundation in knowledge, theory, attitude, and awareness that are essential prerequisites for learning feminist executive skills.

Executive Skills

Cleghorn and Levin (1973) define executive skills as the ability to "influence the family to demonstrate the way it functions," and the ability to "influence the family's sequences of transactions so as to alter the way it functions" (p. 441). Tomm and Wright (1979) emphasize that executive skills are best understood as consisting of two components. The first is the actual overt intervention a therapist makes, and the second is the ability of the therapist to use her or his "own emotional reactions constructively by channeling them into specific therapeutic activity" (p.229).

In a feminist approach to family therapy it is extremely important that the therapist be active, directive, and competent. At the same time, however, these skills should be used to influence all members of the family to enter into a collaborative relationship with the therapist, thus minimizing hierarchy.

In a feminist-informed family therapy, as previously noted, it is also vitally important for both the therapist *and* the family to be able to analyze or place their situation within a larger social frame. Such a view sensitizes family members to the impact of the uneven distribution of power and privilege on men and women and the kinds of relationships they form. In this regard, executive skills are consistently directed at reallocating power.

Tomm and Wright's (1979) inclusion of the affective component of executive skills is of particular importance to a feminist approach. Much of family therapy, and in particular structural and strategic approaches, emphasize highly instrumental problem-solving while minimizing the importance of affect in facilitating change. In an attempt to re-integrate and reevaluate emotion and its usefulness in the change process, feminist executive skills should include the ability both to elicit and share emotional responses. It is the affect aroused by a feminist rethinking of the roles, relationships, and decision making patterns within the family which motivates much of the action in the therapy process.

Intervention Model

The following model of feminist family therapy is outlined in terms of specific perceptual/conceptual and executive skills which the therapist may employ. Although many of the skills are actually used throughout therapy, in the interests of clarity they have been divided according to the phase in which they are most important and most useful. The following three phases are each presented with their relevant perceptual/conceptual and executive skills: I. Developing and maintaining a working alliance between family and therapist, II. Defining the problem, and III. Facilitating change.

TRAINING AND SUPERVISION IN A FEMINIST MODEL

Content and Teaching Methods

Training in a feminist model is similar to traditional family therapy training in that many of the same teaching methods may be used. What distinguishes feminist-informed training is its specific feminist content and its use of training processes which are isomorphic to feminist-informed therapy. This relationship between training and therapy has been elaborated elsewhere (Haley, 1976, 1980; Liddle, 1982; Liddle & Saba, 1982; Minuchin & Fishman, 1981). The way in which therapy is taught is particularly important in feminist training, where more positive and less oppressive attitudes toward women, and an understanding of power and gender roles must be taught by example as well as theory.

The goal of a feminist-informed training program is the acquisition of the perceptual/conceptual and executive skills presented in Tables 1, 2, and 3. Because sexist thinking is so pervasive in our society, feminist-based perceptual/conceptual skills cannot adequately be taught simply as a part of the supervisory process. An important first step in learning feminist-informed therapy is a critical study of women's position in society

TABLE 1

Skills for Developing and Maintaining a Working Alliance
Between Family and Therapist

DEVELOPING AND MAINTAINING A WORKING ALLIANCE BETWEEN FAMILY AND THERAPIST

a) Perceptual/Conceptual Skills

— Appreciate the heavy load of responsibility which women carry for family well-being and recognize feelings of guilt and responsibility which women in particular feel when family problems develop.
— Realize that both men and women are victims of gender role socialization and develop a non-blaming attitude towards the socialized behavior of both genders.
— Recognize the importance of joining strongly with men to ensure their participation in a therapy which asks them to give up their privileged position in exchange for unfamiliar benefits.
— Appreciate the value of egalitarian (non-hierarchical) relationships both in the marital relationship and between therapist and family.
— Appreciate the need for an explicit contract which details the expectations and goals of therapy as well as the mutual roles and responsibilities of therapist and family, in the interest of demystifying therapy and reducing hierarchy between the therapist and family.
— Recognize the value of therapist self disclosure for normalizing gender role difficulties and for reducing hierarchy in the therapist's relationship with the family.
— Recognize that therapeutic competence can be established by self assuredness without the need to "take charge" in an authoritarian manner.

b) Executive Skills

— Define the therapeutic alliance as one in which the therapist and the family members have equal status in terms of their responsibility and capability for problem resolution.
— Avoid defining or reacting to the family as "resistant" as this defines the therapist as "expert" and sets an adversarial and competitive tone to the working alliance.
— Negotiate with the family, as equal partners, for what the goals of therapy will be, how long therapy will last, and what particular strategies or interventions are permissible.
— Selectively use self disclosure and self reference in order to empha-

size the commonality of sex role problems, and to de-emphasize the therapist as a neutral or final authority.

— Overtly influence all members of the family toward a more equitable distribution of costs and benefits of family membership.

— Communicate that an important aspect of therapy is to help the family recognize the negative effects of sex role socialization, where they exist, and to explore behavioral alternatives.

TABLE 2

Skills for Defining the Problem

DEFINING THE PROBLEM

a) Perceptual/Conceptual Skills

— Recognize power inequities between husbands and wives as a major dynamic in family problems, and analyze marital relationships in terms of unequal access to influence, control, choice, resources, opportunity, and status.

— Understand the reciprocal relationship between power inequities in marriage and in society, i.e., that the devaluation of women in educational, religious, political, and economic institutions is reflected in and reinforced by their secondary status in marriage.

— Know the theory and research which detail the pervasive negative effects of traditional gender roles on women, men, children, family structure, and interpersonal behavior and relationships.

— Evaluate women positively, including recognizing their strengths and competencies and valuing the important work women do in families.

— Recognize how traditional gender roles reinforce power inequities between men and women and thus contribute to family problems. This recognition should include an understanding of how gender role behavior is taught and maintained in the family.

— Recognize that traditional child rearing arrangements frequently contribute to dysfunctional family structures.

— Appreciate the importance of individual as well as family well-being and recognize that family well-being is oppressive to women when it is accomplished at the expense of their own self-development.

— In assigning meaning to family behaviors, recognize how they contribute to a maintenance of the power structure, and to the continuation of women's traditional role as chief nurturer and caretaker of the family.

—Define family problems in terms of power differentials and stereotyped expectations and behaviors.

b) Executive Skills

—Observe family dynamics for those ideas, behaviors, and interactional sequences which support and maintain power inequities or stereotypic gender roles.
—Assist the family to assess costs and benefits to each individual family member and to the system as a whole of the allocation of roles and responsiblities.
—Determine whether roles result from genuine negotiation and represent the most equitable way to maintain individual and system needs, or reflect instead an unexamined response to social expectations.
—Encourage each family member to share their unique view of the problem, while validating and supporting the *affective* as well as rational components of each member's presentation.
—Make explicit statements or ask questions regarding the impact of context, tradition, or socialization on the problem(s) as defined by the family. (e.g., "What is it about the way women are raised that encourages Mom to feel guilty and unsure about her ability to be a good mother?")
—Reframe or challenge, where appropriate, the family's definition of problems to include the impact of sexism, patriarchical structures, or gender bias.
—Resist overt and covert pressure from the family to assume an "expert" role or to hear the major responsibility for change during therapy.

TABLE 3

Skills for Facilitating Change

FACILITATING CHANGE

a) Perceptual/Conceptual Skills

—Identify stereotypical role behavior as it occurs in the session.
—Recognize the political dimension of therapy and the potential for family therapy to inadvertently reinforce traditional gender roles (Jacobson, 1983).
—Recognize the validity of women's world views and perceptions of reality. These perceptions, growing out of their unique life experience as women, are frequently different from men's.

and in the family. This can best be accomplished through an academic course dealing with feminist theory and issues. Ideally, such a course would be oriented to family therapists and taught by a feminist family systems therapist who could help trainees integrate the linear aspects of feminist thinking with the circularity of family systems thinking. However, in the absence of such a specialized course, an introductory course in women's studies or in feminist theory could provide a similar foundation. It is important for trainees to be exposed to feminist theory from a wide range of disciplines so that they may challenge their own culturally prescribed notions of normality, health, appropriate gender roles, and desirable therapeutic outcomes.

The following content areas are specifically recommended for study: the historical and religious roots of gender inequity; feminist analyses of the masculine assumptions underlying philosophical and scientific theories; feminist analyses of the family and of the institutions of marriage and motherhood; the process and effects of gender role socialization; the psychology of women; economic issues such as paid and unpaid work, pensions for women, the gross overrepresentation of women in poverty statistics and on welfare roles, the effect of capitalism and competitive economics on the family; issues related to violence against women such as rape, incest, wife abuse, and pornography; women's health issues such as menopause, aging, abortion, overmedication with psychotropic drugs and unnecessary surgery; an examination of alternative life styles for women such as lesbianism, singleness, single parenting, and childlessness; critiques of traditional psychotherapy as oppressive to women; the principles of feminist therapy; and the small but growing literature which deals specifically with feminist issues in family therapy. (See Appendices A and B for Annotated Bibliography and Background Reading.)

This type of course usually causes heightened awareness of the trainees' own socialization, gender biases, and experiences of oppression. Such awareness may be further encouraged through small group discussions and through requesting that trainees keep a personal journal for the duration of the course.

Class discussions present a special challenge to the instructor in this type of course since the material tends to be emotionally evocative. Discussions must be well monitored so that they do not degenerate into blaming sessions and so that a positive action-oriented atmosphere is maintained. As women first become aware of the facts of their oppression, it is not unusual for them to become intensely angry (Josofowitz, 1980). It is essential for an instructor to validate female trainees' anger when it occurs and to help them to use it as a mobilizing force toward assertive action in their lives and in the therapy they provide, rather than assuming an angry victim role. As male trainees first become aware of their privileged position in society and of their complicity in the oppression of women, their first reaction is often defensiveness, followed by guilt (Josofowitz, 1980). Validation of these feelings is imperative to help male trainees move beyond defensiveness to a new evaluation of women and an acceptance of partnership in fighting oppression.

When a class or supervisory group is composed of both male and female trainees, instances of the usual male-female power differential often occur spontaneously within the group itself. For example, even when males comprise a very small segment, they often will dominate discussion while women often lack confidence in, and hesitate to communicate their ideas. Men frequently will interrupt, while women will politely defer to them. So insidious is this process that, unless they are alert, even instructors may find themselves giving greater attention to male input than to female. The instructor has a unique opportunity to identify such processes as they occur and to use them to demonstrate feminist concepts. As trainees express feelings about their interactions, they experience a highly impactful and immediate lesson about the power of gender role socialization. Once trainees have achieved the awareness of women's oppression they have a cognitive foundation upon which to base executive skills.

Training in feminist executive skills may proceed simultaneously with that in perceptual/conceptual skills. The supervisor may use typical family therapy training methods such as roleplaying, analyzing videotaped sessions, live supervision, pre- and post-session discussions, and feedback. Examining videotaped therapy sessions through an interactional lens and then through a feminist lens enables therapists to see the differences and similarities between the two and to plan interventions which integrate both. Reviewing videotapes also provides an opportunity for the instructor/supervisor to challenge trainees' stereotypical thinking and behavior, and to present alternatives.

Live supervision, particularly, is useful for teaching feminist perspectives and skills. The supervisor may direct the therapist's attention to underlying power and gender issues, and coach the therapist to challenge the family's stereotypic expectations and behaviors. When there is a team present, the "Greek Chorus" (Papp, 1980) may be used to elevate and empower women by validating their perspective and feelings, providing support in taking firm positions, encouraging self-development, and applauding efforts to take less responsibility for the family. Such live supervision should be feminist in nature, in that peer observers work as an equalitarian team. Rather than developing all interventions, it is the supervisor's responsibility to stimulate discussion of the immediate case by asking the team members' opinions, generating an atmosphere open to creative ideas and suggestions, and helping each team member to become an active part of the supevisory process. This involvement includes sharing responsibility for phoning in interventions which have been discussed and agreed upon by the team.

The Supervisory Relationship

The relationship between supervisor and trainee is a crucial element in the training program, and one which should embody the feminist values and behaviors which the therapist is learning. The major characteristics of this relationship are the minimization of hierarchy and the use of social analysis.

Minimizing Hierarchy. Hierarchy may be minimized in the following ways:

(a) *Contracting.* Although contracting also is used in traditional family therapy training its purpose is somewhat different in a feminist training approach. Here contracting is used to minimize the hierarchy between supervisor and therapist by stipulating shared responsibility for change and learning. The contract becomes a vehicle for negotiating the roles of both supervisor and trainee. At the beginning of training, the supervisor works with each therapist to specify goals, objectives, areas of improvement and ways in which the supervisor can be most useful. The responsibility for the therapist's learning is shared equally by supervisor and therapist, with the supervisor as active as the therapist, but not more so. The supervisor and therapist look at training as a joint venture and the contract is used to underscore this attitude.

(b) *Evaluation.* Hierarchy is also minimized via shared responsibility for evaluation. The learning goals and objectives outlined in the contract become a criteria by which progress can be measured. During and following training, therapists will discuss their own progress and receive and offer feedback from other trainees regarding each one's achievement. As an equal partner in this process the supervisor is also evaluated in terms of his/her effectiveness in helping the trainees to meet their goals.

Feedback is given in an atmosphere where trainees' unique capabilities, individual strengths, and competencies are valued and built upon. One responsibility of the supervisor is to challenge respectfully any stereotypic behavior and to encourage more balanced, androgynous skills. One way to empower a female trainee is to challenge passive, diffident, overly polite behavior. Encouraging her to be active (Caust, Libow, & Raskin, 1981), while also displaying empathy validates traditional female behavior while fostering growth in an instrumental direction. Encouraging expressions of feeling, self-disclosure, warmth, empathy and intuition in male trainees while still appreciating an active, directive therapeutic posture promotes the widening of behavioral repertoires. It is important, then, for supervisors to push both male and female trainees to explore areas of technique, style, and attitude beyond the traditional while

still validating those traditional behaviors which are effective, useful, and positive.

(c) *Use of Language.* Therapists' questions are encouraged, respected and responded to with clear, uncomplicated language and ideas. Such clarity reduces power and status differentials and facilitates learning.

The supervisor, aware of gender bias implicit in our culture, is careful to avoid sexist language and encourages trainees to be equally aware. For example, referring to women clients or therapists as "girls," attending to a woman's appearance rather than her intelligence or competence, and using derogatory labels in regard to female clients, such as "castrating," demeans female clients and trainees alike.

Social Analysis. Social analysis by the trainee and supervisor clarifies and politicizes a therapeutic issue. For example, a supervisor might say, "You're being too polite with these clients. As women we've been taught to be passive, polite, and not to challenge other's ideas or values. But this often isn't useful to us either as women or therapists. Direct your couple to talk to one another rather than asking them so politely to do so. This models an active and competent woman." Building a cognitive bridge between therapist behavior and traditional socialization empowers therapists while teaching them to make broader political connections for themselves and their clients. Such social analysis is all the more powerful when accompanied by appropriate self-disclosure by the supervisor regarding the effect of his/her socialization on his/her therapeutic style.

Social analysis also should take into consideration the gender issues implicit between supervisor and therapist. As Okun (1983) has stated, "gender issues are inevitable in processes of family systems therapy and supervision, and these require primary consideration in establishing and implementing the training curriculum" (p. 45). A major gender issue is the possibility of the supervisor-trainee relationship falling into destructive traditional patterns, as indicated in several ways: submissive or seductive behavior in women; a patronizing or seductive attitude in men; male trainees not taking female supervisors seriously; male therapist's ideas, behaviors, and progress valued above those women (Okun, 1983). Social analysis may be used to make connections between those incidents and traditional attitudes and behaviors supported in society.

CONCLUSION

We have presented a model of feminist family therapy and supervision designed to promote a more gender-sensitive approach to working with families. This approach provides family therapists with an expanded lens through which to view families, and encourages greater role flexibility, equality, and choices for all family members. The supervisor who employs this model is responding to recent feminist critiques of family therapy by pointing the field as well as his/her trainees in a new direction—one which will require both courage and commitment.

REFERENCES

Avis, J. M. (1985). The politics of functional family therapy: A feminist critique. *Journal of Marital and Family Therapy* (in press).

Caust, B. L., Libow, J. A., & Raskin, P. A. (1981). Challenges and promises of training women as family systems therapists. *Family Process, 22,* 439-447.

Cleghorn, J. M., & Levin, S. (1973). Training family therapists by setting learning objectives. *American Journal of Orthopsychiatry, 43* (3), 439-446.

Feldman, L. (1982). Sex roles and family dynamics. In F. Walsh (Ed.), *Normal family processes.* New York: Guilford Press.

Gilbert, L. A. (1980). Feminist therapy. In A. M. Brodsky & R. Hare-Mustin (Eds.), *Women and psychotherapy: An assessment of research and practice.* New York: Guilford Press.

Gurman, A. S. & Klein, M. H. (1984). The family: An unconscious male bias in behavioral treatment? In E. Blechman (Ed.), *Behavior modification with women.* New York: Guilford Press.

Haley, J. (1976). *Problem-solving therapy.* San Francisco, CA: Jossey-Bass.

Haley, J. (1980). *Leaving home: The therapy of disturbed young people.* New York: McGraw Hill.

Hare-Mustin, R. T. (1978). A feminist approach to family therapy. *Family Process, 17,* 181-194.

Hare-Mustin, R. T. (1979). Family therapy and sex role stereotypes. *The Counseling Psychologist, 8* (1), 31-32.

Hartsock, N. (1975). Fundamental feminism: Process and perspective. *Quest: A Feminist Quarterly, 2* (2), 32-43.

Hoffman, L. (1981). *Foundations of family therapy.* New York: Basic Books.

Ivey, A. E. (1971). *Microcounseling: Innovations in interviewing training.* Springfield: Thomas.

Jacobson, N. S. (1983). Beyond empiricism: The politics of marital therapy. *The American Journal of Family Therapy, 11* (2), 11-24.

James, K. & McIntyre, D. (1983). The reproduction of families: The social role of family therapy. *Journal of Marital and Family Therapy, 9* (2), 119-129.

Josofowitz, N. (1980). *Paths to power.* Reading, MA: Addison-Wesley.

Klein, M. H. (1976). Feminist concepts of therapy outcome. *Psychotherapy: Theory, Research, and Practice, 13,* 89-95.

Kolbenschlag, M. (1979). *Kiss sleeping beauty good-bye.* New York: Bantam.

Libow, J. A., Raskin, P. A., & Caust, B. (1982). Feminist and family systems therapy: Are they irreconcilable? *The American Journal of Family Therapy, 10* (3), 3-12.

Liddle, H. (1982). Family therapy training: Current issues, future themes. *International Journal of Family Therapy 4,* 31-97.

Liddle, H. A., & Saba, G. W. (1982). On teaching family therapy at the introductory level: A conceptual model emphasizing a pattern which connects training and therapy. *Journal of Marital and Family Therapy, 8* (1).

Miller, L. A. (1983). Feminism, families and family therapy. Presentation at American Association for Marriage and Family Therapy. Washington, D. C.

Minuchin, S. & Fishman, C. (1981). *Techniques of family therapy.* Cambridge, Mass.: Harvard University Press.

Okun, B. F. (1983). Gender issues of family systems therapists. In B. Okun & S. T. Gladdings (Eds.), *Issues in training marriage and family therapists.* Ann Arbor, MI: ERIC/CAPS.

Papp, P. (1980). The Greek Chorus and other techniques of family therapy. *Family Process, 19* (1), 45-57.

Rice, D. G., & Rice, J. K. (1977). Non-sexist "marital" therapy. *Journal of Marriage and Family Counseling, 3,* 3-10.

Seidler-Feller, D. (1976). Process and power in couples psychotherapy: A feminist view. *Voices,* Fall, 67-71.

Rowbotham, S. (1973). *Woman's consciousness, man's world.* Middlesex: Penguin.

Thorne, B., & Yalom, M. (Eds.)(1983). *Rethinking the family: Some feminist questions.* New York: Longman.

Tomm, K. M., & Wright, L. M. (1979). Training in family therapy: Perceptual, conceptual and executive skills. *Family Process, 18,* 227-250.

Wheeler, D. (1983). Feminism's treatment of women in the family: Implications for family therapy. (Unpublished Manuscript).

APPENDIX A

KEY RESOURCES IN FEMINIST FAMILY THERAPY

*Annotated Bibliography**

Avis, J.M. (In press). The politics of functional family therapy: A feminist critique. *Journal of Marital and Family Therapy.*
This paper examines the political processes and gender biases inherent in functional family therapy. It argues that this model of family therapy subtly reinforces traditional gender roles in both family and therapist and examines the implications of this bias.

Caust, B.L., Libow, J.A. and Raskin, P.A. (1981). Challenges and promises of training women as family systems therapists. *Family Process, 20,* 439-447.
The authors discuss the challenges of family therapy for female clinicians. Included are such topics as expressing authority and power, countertransference, sexual politics of supervision, role models, boundary issues, and the feminine role. The authors suggest that the female family therapist can experience growth beyond traditional behavior, and empowerment as a competent woman when a feminist orientation to the profession is employed.

Feldman, L. (1982). Sex role and family dynamics. In F. Walsh (Ed.), *Normal family processes.* New York: Guilford Press.
This chapter combines research findings with family theory in a thought-provoking discussion of the negative effects of traditional gender roles on all family members as well as on family structure and functioning. Implications for family therapists are discussed.

Gluck, N.R., Dannefer, E. & Miles, K. (1980). Women in families. In E.A. Carter and M. McGoldrick (Eds.), *The family life cycle: A framework for family therapy.* New York: Gardner Press.
This chapter examines some of the changes that have occurred in the lives of women over the past 15 years and how these changes are affecting women as they move through the family life cycle. The stages in the life cycle addressed here include the unattached young adult, the newly formed family, the family with young children, adolescent children, the launching stage, older-aged and divorced women.

Gurman, A.S. & Klein, M. (1984). Marriage and the family: An unconscious male bias in behavioral treatment? In E.A. Blechman (Ed.), *Behavior modification with women.* New York: Guilford Press.
This chapter clearly and persuasively critiques the unconscious gender bias inherent in the philosophy and practice of behavioral marital and family therapy. The authors argue that clarification and acknowledgement by the therapist of their own personal and professional values is essential to avoid this bias in practice.

Hare-Mustin, R.T. (1978). A feminist approach to family therapy. *Family Process, 17,* 181-194.
This important article describes the ways in which family therapists who are aware of their own biases and those of the family can change sexist patterns through applying feminist principles through the therapeutic contract, shifting tasks in the family, communication, generational boundaries, relabeling deviance, modeling, and therapeutic alliances.

Hare-Mustin, R.T. (1979). Family therapy and sex role stereotypes. *The Counseling Psychologist, 8,* 31-32.

---

*Also appears in Piercy, F. and Sprenkle, D. (In press). *Family therapy sourcebook.* New York: Guilford.

Primarily a summary of her 1978 paper, Hare-Mustin critiques techniques of family therapy and recommends knowledge, skills and attitudes necessary for family therapists to confront sex role stereotypes in their own lives and those of their clients.

Hare-Mustin, R.T. (1980). Family therapy may be dangerous for your health. *Professional Psychology, 11,* 935-938.

Hare-Mustin points out the dangers involved when therapists give priority to the good of the family, thereby negating the best interests of individual family members (most often women). She also suggests that most family therapists accept the traditional model of the family and make this model their goal. This often fosters stereotyped roles and other behaviors which impinge upon the well-being of women.

Jacobson, N.S. (1983). Beyond empiricism: The politics of marital therapy. *American Journal of Family Therapy, 11,* 11-24.

This article provides an excellent discussion of the political (i.e., power) issues implicit in therapy in general and behavioral marital therapy in particular. Jacobson identifies the processes through which traditional values and roles oppressive to women are inadvertently reinforced and makes specific recommendations for changing them.

James, K. & McIntyre, D. (1983). The reproduction of families: The social role of family therapy? *Journal of Marital and Family Therapy, 9,* 119-129.

The authors challenge family therapy's failure to respond to recent critical analyses of the family as well as its failure to consider the socio-economic-political contexts of family functioning. They examine systems theory's limitations (i.e., locating family dysfunction entirely within family structure), problems inherent in the institution of motherhood, and the social role of the family therapist. An excellent discussion is included on several key issues.

Libow, J.A., Raskin, P.A. and Caust, B.L. (1982). Feminist and family systems therapy: Are they irreconcilable? *American Journal of Family Therapy, 10,* 3-12.

This article identifies the differences and similarities between feminist and family therapy, both in theory and technique. Differences include views of causality, locus of change, insight and the use of power. The two frameworks share techniques of modeling and reframing, contextual concepts of pathology and emphasis on behavioral change. Further integration of the two frameworks is encouraged.

Margolin, G., Fernandez, V., Talovic, S. & Onorato, R. (1983). Sex role considerations and behavioral marital therapy: Equal does not mean identical. *Journal of Marital and Family Therapy, 9,* 131-145.

This worthwhile paper examines the advantages and disadvantages of behavioral marital therapy (BMT) in terms of the way in which it treats men and women. The authors identify a variety of ways in which BMT gives contradictory messages regarding sex role issues and make recommendations for how BMT can become more sensitive to these issues as well as more flexible in handling them.

Okun, B.F. (1983). Gender issues of family systems therapists. In B.F. Okun and S.T. Gladding (Eds.), *Issues in training marriage and family therapists.* Ann Arbor, Mich.: ERIC/CAPS.

This well-written article provides a good introduction to gender issues in both the training of family therapists and the practice of family therapy. It raises a number of key issues relevant to all family therapists regardless of theoretical orientation, such as the impact of gender differences and socialization on the supervisory relationship as well as on therapist's attitudes and behavior.

Riche, M. (1984). The systemic feminist. *Family Therapy Networker, 8(3)* 43-44.

This short, well-written article describes how the author reconciles apparent contradictions between feminism and family therapy in her own practice. The author uses case studies to illustrate her feminist approach to therapy both before and after she began applying systems concepts. This article would be particularily useful for the practicing clinician.

Simon, R. (1984). From ideology to practice: The Women's Project in Family Therapy. *Family Therapy Networker, 8(3),* 28-32, 38-40.

Richard Simon interviews the four organizers of the Women's Project in Family Therapy: Betty Carter, Olga Silverstein, Peggy Papp, and Marianne Walters. In this provocative interview, these leaders candidly discuss their own experiences with sexism, the development of the Women's Project, and ways they are implementing their feminist ideology in family therapy.

APPENDIX B

BACKGROUND READING

Bernard, J. (1975). *The future of motherhood.* New York: Penguin Books.
Bernard, J. (1982). *The future of marriage* (2nd ed.). New Haven: Yale University Press.
Brodsky, A. M. & Hare-Mustin, R. T. (Eds.). (1980). *Women and psychotherapy.* NY: Guilford.
Brownmiller, S. (1975). *Against our will: Men, women and rape.* NY: Simon and Schuster.
Chesler, P. (1972). *Women and madness.* New York: Doubleday.
Chodorow, N. (1978). *The reproduction of mothering.* Berkeley: University of California Press.
Dworkin, A. (1974). *Woman Hating.* NY: E. P. Dutton.
Ehrenreich, B. & English, D. (1979). *For her own good: 150 years of the experts' advice to women.* Garden City, NY: Anchor Books.
Eisenstein, H. (1983). *Contemporary feminist thought.* Boston, MA: G. K. Hall.
Gilligan, C. (1982). *In a different voice.* Cambridge, MA: Harvard University Press.
Gornick, V. & Moran, B. K. (1971). *Women in sexist society.* NY: Basic Books.
Jaggar, A. M. & Struhl, P. R. (1978). *Feminist frameworks,* NY: McGraw-Hill.
Kolbenschlag, M. (1979). *Kiss sleeping beauty good-bye.* New York: Bantam.
Miller, J. B. (1976). *Toward a new psychology of women.* Boston, MA: Beacon Press.
Morgan, R. (1970). *Sisterhood is powerful.* NY: Vintage Books.
Tavris, D. & Offir, C. (1977). *The longest war: Sex differences in perspective.* New York: Harcourt, Brace, Jovanovich.

An Intensive Training Experience:
A Six Day Post Graduate Institute Model

Florence Kaslow

ABSTRACT. A six-day intensive training model is presented which provides a post-graduate workshop experience for practicing family therapy
professionals. The present article describes and discusses the nature and
content of this intensive workshop experience.

Once a therapist completes his/her graduate or professional school
and/or Family Institute training, most additional education is acquired
through reading professional books and journals and attending symposia
or workshops at conferences. Usually these run from one hour to two
days and opportunities to share intensively what has been transpiring in
the areas of one's clinical practice, professional growth and therapeutic
"stuck" spots are nil to minimal. A six-day intensive training model was
designed to provide such an opportunity in a teaching—learning—sharing
environment constructed specifically for this purpose. From the feedback
received from the participants in the first three such workshops, it has
fulfilled its objectives.

This article will describe, highlight and analyze the nature and content
of the Institute and try to articulate the major elements that contribute to
its apparent success. The observations presented, of course, are biased,
but reflect well the enthusiasm this model has generated, based on feedback from participants, and their recommendations to colleagues to attend
future similar events at the Florida Couples and Family Institute.

THE TRAINING MODEL

Time Frame

The workshops are designed to run for six consecutive days from 9AM
to 4PM with an hour for lunch. This was done to enhance the continuity

Florence Kaslow, Ph.D., is Director of the Florida Couples and Family Institute, Northwood
Medical Center, Suite 204, 2617 North Flagler Drive, West Palm Beach, FL 33407, and is in independent practice in West Palm Beach, Florida. She is also an Adjunct Professor, Department of
Psychiatry, Duke University, Durham, North Carolina, and former Editor of the *Journal of Marital
and Family Therapy.*

and intensity of the experience—drawing on the findings gleaned from the human potential movement that marathon training events tend to diminish barriers to involvement and to promote self disclosure (Shutz, 1967), unfreezing, and openness to new learning. This fact has been verified by our experience; all participants become deeply engaged with each other, the trainers, the content and their own self as central to their learning process and their universe as a therapist/supervisor/teacher and/or trainer.

The Setting and Ambiance

The Florida Couples and Family Institute is situated in the Palm Beaches in a suite of offices in a medical complex. The main classroom is cheerfully decorated, with comfortable couches and a formica table that doubles for writing or dining. This room houses videotape equipment and accommodates ten people. Another smaller adjacent room also has soft couches and is used as a reading or study room. There is a desk for anyone wishing to write during breaks or lunch hours. All of the offices in the Institute suite abound with marital and family therapy books and journals which participants are encouraged to borrow.

All Institutes have been held between November and March when the climate in Southern Florida is lovely. Several days staff and participants are likely to bring lunches and picnic in the scenic lakeside park across from the office. This too facilitates the getting better acquainted and establishment of mutuality and trust. The other days everyone packs into cars to drive to any one of a good assortment of classy and/or nice but inexpensive nearby restaurants to sample regional specialties. The lovely palm tree lined boulevards enhance the relaxation and splendor of the environs.

Participants have come from near (Palm Beaches, Ft. Lauderdale, Miami) and far (South Africa, Israel, North Carolina). Each workshop group has been comprised of Americans and people from abroad, giving the group a sophisticated, multicultural coloration. It has also meant that the majority of those attending need housing accommodations. We have worked out special rates and arrangements with a nearby hotel and motel, and at each event, all of the out-of-town participants have stayed at the same facility. Generally they have chipped in together and shared car rentals, gone swimming together at the hotel pool, and often decided to have dinner and spend part of the evening together—going over the events and challenges of the day and often building wonderful friendships. Several times people have roomed together. For example, earlier this year we teamed up a psychology professor from the University of Pretoria with a psychiatry resident from Duke University. They became and remain good friends. Those who commute realize they are missing the special lure of recreated dormitory living, adult style, and sometimes also decide to share the more total experience by staying at the hotel or motel.

Staff also join them for dinner and evening festivities whenever possible. Once during the institute my family and I hosted a reception at our condominium in honor of the participants, and institute staff and faculty. This too enhances the collegial nature of the endeavor and the "family" aura of the entire event. We truly work and play together; this symbolically represents also a theme in the workshop of the importance of families achieving a vital balance between work and play, formality and informality, closeness and privacy.

WORKSHOP CONTENT AND FORMAT

Two of the workshops have focused on "Advanced Marital and Family Therapy". The third centered on "Advanced Supervision and Staff Training". Only the Institute revolving around the first topic will be discussed here to illustrate the model.

Preparation

When participants enroll they are sent a two page tentative syllabus so they can begin thinking about and preparing for the workshop. Since most travel quite a distance (they are investing quite a large chunk of time and money in the registration fee, airfare, hotel and their allied expenses), they expect a high quality experience, and this is what we seek to provide from the moment that they register.

Each person is invited and encouraged to bring a videotape of their work to present for discussion and consultation. Since not everyone working outside of major training centers has access to taping equipment, and tapes made in foreign countries are often not compatible with our equipment, other options are also suggested (e.g., written family case summaries and/or audiotapes). We xerox the case records so all participants have them to follow in their case book and to take home with other materials distributed to them.

Course of the Workshop

On *Day 1,* by design, I spend the entire day orienting the group and trying to facilitate the evolution of cohesion and esprit de corp. Members spend a good deal of time introducing themselves—telling about their professional setting, work responsibilities and philosophy of family therapy. They also share, albeit cautiously at first, a little about their families of origin and families of creation, as well as their professional extended family. They indicate why they decided to come to this particular workshop and what their personal goals are, from this involvement.

Next we look at common themes in their objectives. Throughout there is an effort to help them feel "safe" in their explorations and revelations.

Being away from a competitive environment or one in which they are expected to be an expert may be heady wine—for here it is safe to say "I don't know," or "that's a concept that eludes me." No one is evaluating performance, nor is the atmosphere conducive to one-upsmanship. What seems to evolve early-on is the sense of embarking on an adventure together. As they tell what it is they would like to learn more about, we refashion the syllabus to accommodate their interests. Since each group is purposely kept small—and ranges from six to ten trainees—such specific tailoring is not difficult. Throughout, participants draw from their collective knowledge and experiences, and exchange ideas—serving as resources for each other and supplementing what the trainers provide.

In the afternoon I begin an in-depth overview of the major theoretical schools of family therapy. Several are covered each day—either by me or on subsequent days by another faculty member with specific expertise in a particular approach and its accompanying techniques. Using my diaclectic model (Kaslow, 1981) as a framework in which to compare, contrast differentiate and integrate the various theoretical approaches, we cover a wide variety of theoretical perspectives and their leading proponents (Kaslow, 1985).

1. Psychodynamic (Ackerman, Beatman & Sherman, 1961)
2. Bowenian (Bowen, 1978)
3. Contextual/Relational (Boszormenyi-Nagy & Spark, 1973)
4. Experiential (Keith & Whitaker, 1981; Napier & Whitaker, 1978; Neill & Kniskern, 1982)
5. Communications/Interpersonal (Satir, 1964)
6. Structural (Minuchin, 1974)
7. Strategic (Fisch, Weakland & Segal, 1982; Haley, 1976; Madanes, 1981)
8. Systemic (Selvini-Palazzoli, Boscolo, Cecchin, Prata, 1978)
9. Problem Solving (Epstein & Bishop, 1981)
10. Behavioral (Jacobson & Margolin, 1979)
11. Diaclectic, Integrative, Multimodal (Duhl & Duhl, 1979; Kaslow, 1981; Lazarus, 1981)

Participants usually are cognizant of most, but not all of the theories. They have not been exposed to all of them in their own terms as well as in comparative relationship to each other. They grapple with this broad articulation and the myriad possibilities this panorama opens up in terms of selecting the specific approach and techniques which seem to have the greatest explanatory and healing power for each family, problem and situation. During the workshop most participants gradually relinquish any totalistic purist commitment to any one way being the best and/or only right way. We reframe their transgression or disloyalty to their favorite "guru" teacher as independent, expansive thinking and the group nurtures this non-ethnocentric thrust.

On *Day 2* we consider various assessment devices. Since we usually cover the major premises of Bowenian systems theory (Bowen, 1978) at this time, I ask everyone to *do your genogram* and briefly go over the symbols utilized in the universal language of genogramming, if they are not all familiar with this (Guerin & Fogarty, 1972). Since this has proven to be one of the most productive and illuminating portions of the training (and of other workshops into which I often incorporate it), I will elaborate my approach in some detail. The reader will note that it builds on some aspects of traditional genogramming but also departs in some significant ways.

About eight or more years ago when I was teaching a family therapy course at Hahnemann Medical University, when I explained the genogram symbols and told my students to draw their family—I inadvertently forgot to say "family of origin" and "start as far back as you remember". When we moved into a discussion of their family trees, what surprised me was that, given the freedom to proceed from an inner directed logic, each person started at the most central and logical place for him/her. Each was amazed to find out later that their classmates drew someone else first; they each realized they put down that person first who was most pivotal in their current universe. Several drew themselves first, others a spouse, parent, grandparent, sibling, or child. Where they began is multi-determined and quite informative.

Since that first "error" I now begin simply by saying "draw your family" and giving no other directions. For me, the genogram has become an excellent personal family projective assessment tool. Once they have depicted their family, we explore such questions as:

Who did you put down first?

What specific significance does that person have to you at this point in time?

If they are surprised at their preoccupation with someone—we pursue this further in terms of:

What unfinished business do you have with this person that you'd like to work through? How might you go about it?

The next sequence of questions might follow the remark,

Take another look at the genogram and see who you failed to include.

People are amazed and sometimes chagrined or puzzled to notice they omitted a sibling, step parent, former spouse who is a parent to their children, or a grandparent. We pursue what this means to them and often strong, negative feelings are evoked. It becomes evident that some individuals include dead former relatives who were important to them and others do not. Often they have not completed the mourning process and I may move into a discussion of Williamson's article on graveside visits to facilitate closure on grief work (Williamson, 1978). This usually has a profound effect as they become conscious of the longings, loss and anger associated with a departed loved one and potentially acquire a new way to personally deal with this and bring to closure an incompletely resolved relationship. On a professional level they absorb awareness of a technique they can incorporate into their clinical practice with others confronted by this dilemma.

Often someone will spontaneously declare "I left my in-laws off" and then rationalize—"You said 'draw my family' and they are part of my spouse's family". Yet it rapidly becomes apparent that others present included their in-laws and that if they are not part of the picture, that the children seem to have descended from one set of grandparents only. When included they often like and respect their in-laws although on occasion this inclusion signifies over-involvement in a distressing negative interaction. What usually emerges are feelings of nonacceptance, rejection, hostility, enmeshment, and detachment, often of long standing, and not dealt with or dealt with insufficiently in their own personal therapy. The processing of the above experiences may provide the impetus for a voyage home or, if they are in therapy, for a multigenerational family therapy session.

A didactic presentation of transgenerational influences is interwoven with or follows the in-depth, profoundly moving experience of working with personal genograms as projective as well as historic documents. We shift levels from experiential to theoretical, from personal to professional, bearing in mind always that the participants have contracted for an intensive training experience and not a treatment marathon. There is however a commitment to the idea that one becomes most cognizant of theory and technique by grappling with them experientially (Kaslow, 1984) in training, therapy and the larger experience of living.

The next series of questions emanate from the core one of:

Who would you like to eliminate?

Amidst startled expressions and anxious giggles—at least several people will erase someone. The less inhibited will scribble them out as small children do. Most frequent on the list of people to be annihilated are nasty ex-spouses, wicked stepmothers and rivalrous siblings. This often leads into a discussion of repressed anger in family relationships and how it sometimes explodes and takes the form of child or spouse abuse, suicide, homicide or running away and cutting off all contact. They are asked to feel and explore their own wellsprings of anger, how they cope with it, and then to identify with the feelings of the abusive, destructive person who is unable to channel the rage constructively and instead acts out violently. Some participants report months later that this segment of the training has given them a much better comprehension of and empathic ability to work with abusive patients and other anti-social family members they treat.

The final section of this voyage into their unique family bonds and cut offs revolves around the query:

Who would you like to add?

Reactions range from a smile at the expansive prospect to misty eyes over a vacuum experienced that cannot be filled. Some want to add a sibling, a spouse or a child. We may explore how this longing can be actualized, considering many options like emotionally adopting a friend or cousin as a sibling, seeking a partner, or rearranging some priorities to have or adopt a child. Others would like to include a parent, grandparent or sibling who died when they were young and who they never had the opportunity to know. Here we again may do some grief work and/or suggest ways of making a psychological and physical pilgrimmage into one's past (e.g., to talk with those who did know them and might be willing to recount their memories). The themes and issues evoked from this genogram exploration permeate the entire training event.

After some more neutral time spent discussing psychodynamic approaches (Ackerman, Beatman & Sherman, 1961) and the intertwining of concern for intrapsychic as well as interpersonal aspects of being in a family, as well as the role of the past and psychic determinism in current family dynamics and functioning, we go on to the concepts of invisible loyalties, entitlement and obligations (Boszormenyi-Nagy & Spark, 1972). Following the rational presentation of this complex material we will again move to a more experiential mode.

Usually I will have a visiting faculty member come in and lead the next segment. In 1984, Sue Fieldman guided the participants through a memory lane trip through a home of their childhood, raising key evocative questions related to:

Who was in the house when you got home from school? What smells do you remember from the kitchen? What were the sleeping arrangements and those about privacy and shared space, opened and closed doors, joint activities, raised argumentative voices, and seating arrangements at mealtime?

Long obscured happy and sad memories resurfaced and all present agreed this poignant fantasy tour constitutes a powerful way to bring about the return of the repressed.

Next, we are likely to review structural (Minuchin, 1974), strategic (Haley 1976, Madanes, 1981) and systemic (Selvini-Palazzoli et al., 1978) approaches, with emphasis on formulating a systemic hypothesis, reframing, establishing clear boundaries, and delivering paradoxical, strategic and/or other here-and-now interventions.

Starting with *day two* participants will be presenting their own previously prepared cases. We attempt to use cases handled from a particular theoretical perspective immediately following the didactic presentation of that approach. It illustrates the theory in action. If there is no case representing a particular philosophy, I may draw vignettes from my practice and/or we may do some spontaneous simulations to illustrate the techniques and their intended impact.

Durings days 3, 4, and 5 we essentially follow a similar format. I'll intersperse the more substantive, carefully delineated approaches like the McMaster Problem Solving Model (Epstein & Bishop, 1981) and the Communications/Brief Therapy Model (Satir, 1964; Fisch et al., 1982) with the Experiential model (Whitaker & Malone, 1981; Napier & Whitaker, 1978). Each approach and its underlaying assumptions are taught utilizing the vocabulary and hopefully the persuasive bent of its adherents.

Guest Lecturers

Initially when people register we ask about their special areas of interest and the patient populations they serve. Based on this, guest faculty are invited. At the 1984 workshop, in addition to Sue Fieldman mentioned earlier, Norma Schulman[2] spoke on hypnotherapy in conjunction with family therapy and Marlys Maury[3] talked about and showed a film on treating the substance abuse family. Gloria Weeks[4] did some of the teaching of Bowenian family therapy, an area in which there was a tremendous amount of interest and to which our South African and Israeli participants have much less exposure than to other theoretical schools. Despite the closeness the core group establishes, they have been receptive to and inclusive of guest faculty and staff.

Closure and Termination

The afternoon of the fifth day is devoted to a diaclectic, integrative model and everyone has a chance to formulate the expansions, shifts and modifications that have occurred for them. Since much bonding has been achieved, the universal, multicultural themes of attachment and separation come to the fore and are processed. Time is spent assessing how what they learned, received and gave met with their aims and expectations. Each is asked to silently think through what they derived that was most beneficial and then to share what they choose to with the group. Often dramatic breakthroughs and "aha" phenomenon are mentioned; others focus on substantive areas of learning that have been enlightening. Trading addresses and hugs usually accompany the goodbyes. In addition to leaving with case books and reprints, everyone gets a certificate for framing and/or continuing education credit.

CONCLUSION

The intensive five- or six-day workshop format provides a unique learning/teaching/sharing opportunity in which seasoned clinicians can shed their barriers and be receptive to becoming more attuned to a variety of different ways of formulating a diagnostic assessment or systemic hypothesis about family dynamics, structure and functioning. They are exposed to assessment devices including paper and pencil scales (e.g., Moos & Moos, 1983; Olson & Portner, 1983) as well as experiential techniques including genogramming, sculpting and the use of family photographs (Kaslow & Friedman, 1977). The experience is structured to include lunches together, some dinners, and an evening reception. In addition, most participants stay in the same hotel or motel and spend part of their free time discussing the readings, the day's events, on both theoretical and personal levels.

We evaluate and modify as we go along, and in the final session. The concensus is that a 36-hour training event held over five or six consecutive days has a much greater emotional and cognitive impact than a 36-hour course spread out over a 12 week semester and broken into 1½-hour classes twice a week or three-hour classes once a week. The richness of working and living together away from family and professional responsibilities and distractions provides a welcome change of pace that fosters immersion in the experience. Recently I have been asked to create a similar format on forthcoming speaking trips to South Africa and Israel because of the unique and compelling appeal of the model. We will also continue to use it in South Florida.

NOTES

1. Sue Fieldman is in private practice in West Hartford, Connecticut and is an adjunct faculty member in the Department of Family Studies at the University of Connecticut in Storrs, Connecticut.

2. Norma Shulman, Ph.D. is a psychologist and family therapist in private practice in West Palm Beach, Florida.

3. Marlys Maury is a drug and alcoholism Counselor at Palm Beach Institute, an in-patient faculty for treating substance abuse that requires involvement for co-dependents.

4. Gloria Weeks, M.S.W., is a staff therapist at the Florida Couples and Family Institute whose orientation has been primarily Bowenian at Syracuse University in the family therapy tract in the School of Social Work.

REFERENCES

Ackerman, N.W. Beatman, F.L. & Sherman, S.N. (1961). *Exploring the base of family therapy.* New York: Family Service Association of America.

Boszormenyi-Nagy, I. & Spark, G. (1973). *Invisible loyalties.* New York: Harper & Row (Reprinted 1984-New York: Brunner/Mazel).

Bowen, M. (1978). *Family therapy in clinical practice.* New York: Jason Aronson.

Duhl, F.J. & Duhl, B.S. (1979). Structured spontaneity; The thoughtful art of integrative family therapy at BFI. *Journal of Marital and Family Therapy, 5,* 59-76.

Epstein, N.B. & Bishop, D.S. (1981). Problem centered systems therapy of the family. In A.S. Gurman & D.P. Kniskern (Eds.), *Handbook of family therapy.* New York: Brunner/Mazel.

Fisch, R., Weakland, J.H. & Segal, L. (1982). *The tactics of change.* San Francisco: Jossey Bass.

Guerin, P. & Fogarty, T. (1972). Study your own family. In A. Ferber, M. Mendelson, & A. Napier (Eds.), *The book of family therapy.* New York: Science House.

Haley, J. (1976). *Problem solving therapy.* San Francisco: Jossey Bass.

Jacobson, N. & Margolin, G. (1979). *Marital therapy.* New York: Brunner/Mazel.

Kaslow, F.W. (1981). A diaclectic approach to family therapy and practice: Selectively and synthesis. *Journal of Marital and Family Therapy, 7,* (3), 345-351.

Kaslow, F.W. (1984). Treatment of marital and family therapists. In F.W. Kaslow (Ed.), *Psychotherapy with psychotherapists.* New York: Haworth Press.

Kaslow, F.W. (1985). Theories of marital and family therapy: A continuum or a smorgasbord? In M. Sussman & S. Steinmetz (Eds.), *Handbook on marriage and the family.* New York: Plenum.

Kaslow, F.W. & Friedman, J. (1977). Utilization of family photos and movies in family therapy. *Journal of Marital and Family Therapy, 3* (1), 19-25.

Keith, D.V. & Whitaker, C.A. (1981). Play therapy: A paradigm for work with families. *Journal of Marital and Family Therapy, 7,* 243-254.

Lazarus, A. (1981). *The practice of multi-modal therapy.* New York: McGraw Hill.

Madanes, C. (1981). *Strategic family therapy.* San Francisco: Jossey Bass.

Minuchin, S. (1974). *Families and family therapy.* Cambridge: Harvard University Press.

Moos, R.H. and Moos, B.S. (1983). Clinical applications of the family environment scale. In E.E. Filsinger (Ed), *Marriage family assessment.* Beverly Hills: Sage Publications.

Napier, A.Y. & Whitaker, C.A. (1978). *The family crucible.* New York: Harper & Row.

Neill, J.R. & Kniskern, D.R. (1982). *From psyche to system: The evolving therapy of Carl Whitaker.* New York: Guilford.

Olson, D.H. & Portner, J. (1983). Family adaptability and cohesion evaluation scales. In E.E. Filsinger (Ed) *Marriage and family assessment.* Beverly Hills: Sage Publications.

Satir, V. (1964). *Conjoint family therapy.* Palo Alto: Science and Behavior Books.

Selvini-Palazzoli, M., Boscolo, L., Cecchin, G., & Prata, G. (1978). *Paradox and counterparadox.* New York: Jason Aronson.

Schutz, W. (1967). *Joy—expanding human awareness.* New York: Grove Press.

Whitaker, C.A. & Malone, T.P. (1981). *The roots of psychotherapy.* New York: Brunner/Mazel.

Williamson, D.S. (1978). New life at the graveyard: A method of therapy for individuation from a dead former parent, *Journal of Marital and Family Therapy, 4,* 93-101.

Family Therapy Supervision: An Integrative Model

James F. Keller
Howard Protinsky

ABSTRACT. The authors present an integrative model of supervision which uses the process of the supervision group to help supervisees become aware of and deal with family-of-origin patterns that may inhibit their therapeutic effectiveness. As this approach is a group supervision model which seeks to understand the supervisory group in a systemic way, the concept of change in supervision is isomorphic to the concept of change in systems family therapy taught in the training program.

Supervision in psychotherapy generally lacks clear boundaries and theoretical structure. The lines are particularly fuzzy around mixing models in supervision and training. For example, there is a lack of clarity regarding a) use of individual supervision methodologies with systemic models of therapy, b) differences among supervision, therapy, and training, c) responsibility of supervisor for supervisee or clients, and d) criteria for more informed choices between models of supervision. Currently there is a surge of interest in supervision and an increase in the number of articles on the subject (e.g., Ard, 1973; Berger and Dammann, 1982; Cormier and Bernard, 1982; Fisher and Keele, 1981; Liddle and Halpin, 1978; Montalvo, 1973; Keller and Protinsky, 1984; Protinsky and Keller, 1984). Most reflect important observations of a largely uncharted frontier, but provide little help in clarifying the issues mentioned above. What is needed is a conscious move toward mapping the territory.

There are a number of ways to chart the territory of family therapy supervision. Reviewing and categorizing the literature helps. It gives us the list of "towns, cities, counties" which are "out there". The next logical step is to begin to construct partial maps with more details of the ways the "towns, cities and counties" can be connected, how they structurally

James F. Keller, Ph.D., is a Professor of Marriage and Family Therapy and Director of the Graduate Training Program in Marriage and Family Therapy, Center for Family Services, Virginia Polytechnic Institute and State University, Blacksburg, VA 24061.

Howard Protinsky, Ph.D., is an Associate Professor of Marriage and Family Therapy at the Center for Family Services at Virginia Polytechnic Institute and State University, Blacksburg, VA 24061.

are related. In other words, we need to construct partial maps for clarifying boundaries around supervision. The purpose of this chapter is to offer one model of family therapy supervision as an example of a partial map. Other approaches to family therapy supervision (e.g., "live", video-taped variations, etc.) are not included in this model.

THEORETICAL BOUNDARY MARKERS

Our integrative model of family therapy supervision has several important boundary markers which may help deal with some of the supervision issues mentioned above. First we assume that clarity and direction can be improved if supervision models are used which are isomorphic with models of therapy taught and practiced in the training program. For example, a group systems model of supervision used with supervisees who practice systemic family therapy (i.e. the supervision model we will discuss) is more isomorphic than an individual, intra-psychically oriented supervision model.

Secondly, we assume that a supervisee's experience within a supervision group (whose members are aware of each supervisee's patterns of fusion and emotional triangling) offers opportunities for supervisees to experience their emotional triangling patterns in a different context. The supervisor's goal is to facilitate the group to interact in nontriangling patterns to increase the probability that the supervisee will be forced to change his/her own fused pattern of interaction. This experience is assumed to provide new dimensions to the supervisee's understanding and ability to manage self when "stuckness" occurs in therapy.

The ultimate goal of supervision, as we see it, is actually a combination of "management of self" and case management methodologies (e.g., techniques for getting "unstuck"). In many supervision approaches a case management methodology is primary, i.e., when a supervisee gets stuck, techniques for getting unstuck are the focus. However, one problem with a sole focus on such techniques is that the supervisees' own recurring patterns of fusion and triangulation may be ignored. On the other end of the continuum, there are personal growth models of supervision which emphasize gains in insight about current patterns of interpersonal behavior and emotional sensitivity. The goal of the insight is not directly to resolve these problems but to develop sensitivity, empathy, and self-monitoring practices. Perhaps because in supervision any indication of behavior that resembles therapy is supposed to be avoided, the growth models are caught in a bind. The growth must be *educative* insight and not *therapeutic* growth. If these boundaries between growth and education are too clearly drawn, the supervision runs the risk of becoming therapy on the one hand or too detached from the actual interaction between the patient/supervisee/supervisor/group on the other. It is our opinion that these problems can best be addressed in a group experience with primary emphasis placed on the group supervision process and secondary emphasis placed on techniques of case management.

These assumptions lay the groundwork for clarifying a partial map for supervision in family therapy. They will now be examined in more detail.

A PARTIAL MAP OF FAMILY THERAPY SUPERVISION

Supervision, historically, has been understood to serve the function of examining and reviewing the supervisee's work. The review process has educative, administrative and supportive goals (Hart, 1982).

We depart from these general goals in a few important ways. First, the primary educative function of our integrative model is not to survey or attempt to incorporate the many diverse approaches to supervision. The most appropriate direction for supervision at this time seems to be toward more theoretical boundary development. We assume that clear theoretical boundaries make for more intelligent adaptation, growth and expansion of various approaches to supervision. We are not suggesting one model to which everyone must subscribe, but the creation of many models whose boundaries are clearly marked and are isomorphic to the therapy practiced.

Another difference of our own model has to do with its definition of "support." Support is defined here as a "stroke and kick." A kick is a response by the supervisor and/or group members which draws attention to and attempts to counter the supervisee's attempts at triangulation. Generally a "kick" is any behavior by the supervisor/group which fosters differentiation and discourages fusion. These statements/behaviors have the effect of raising intensity and pushing ("kicking") the supervisee to expand options for coping with patterns of fusion. The most favorable context for these "kicks" is one in which "strokes" are prevalent. By "strokes" we mean an emphasis on strengths (e.g., reporting examples of differentiation that occur in group interaction, creating a supportive context, and positively connoting supervisee's attempts at triangulating). To always "kick" a supervisee puts too much emphasis on change. To accept everything with strokes puts too little emphasis on growth. Again. a "both-and" philosophy is warranted.

In order to organize the wealth of data that is offered by the interactions within the supra-system of supervisor, supervisory group, therapist and family, a theoretical model is needed. We have employed the Bowen (1978) and Adler/Toman (Toman, 1976) models to lend understanding to the patterns of interaction within such a system.

Our integrative model of supervision in family therapy incorporates the supervision group as a fundamental component of the entire process. Supervisees and supervisors are a working group. This structure is isomorphic to the therapist and family as a working group. During the group supervision period, one supervisee makes a case presentation from case notes and then shows portions of a videotape with the client family. The supervisee's interactions with the group are often discussed as an integral part of the supervision process. Examples from the videotape of healthy differentiation of self from the client family's entangling emotional triangles are compared with similar interactions of the supervisee within the supervisory group. Expressions of emotional fusion from the tape are linked with comparable interactions within the group. Lack of boundary definition from the supervisee within the group (and prior to that within his/her family of origin) can provide clues for examining similar patterns within the therapy session.

What is usually observed during a case presentation in the group is the activation of supervisee's cognitive beliefs and/or emotional responses by a familiar pattern long since learned in his/her family of origin. For example, the supervisee may maneuver a third person in the group into a triangle to drain off his/her anxiety, just as he/she did as a child. Typical expressions of such movement include "pleading eyes", a hesitant voice, expressions of confusion and changing the topic of conversation. These communication expressions are not as likely to appear in one-to-one supervision models, and self-reports are unlikely to catch this level of emotional fusion.

Group members frequently will challenge the supervisee's maneuver toward fusion by refusing to talk about the changed topic, by looking away from the "pleading eyes", by verbalizing what appears to be a nonverbal communication demand, by allowing the supervisee to struggle through an anxious experience assuming actively that he/she can handle the direct challenge. The group experience raises intensity for the supervisees, and it is this very intensity that is presumed to enable the supervisee to expand his/her repertoire of interactional responses to anxiety. This concept of change is isomorphic to the construct of change in systems family therapy taught in our training program.

Another supervision strategy includes paradoxically encouraging the supervisee to provoke emotional triangles during the presentation of case material. Paradoxical supervisory techniques makes it more difficult to continue repeating the triangling pattern and can raise the intensity level which increases the probability of new or different options for more direct communication. We expect these experiences to have carry-over impact when the supervisee conducts therapy.

Our approach is a departure from typical educational models of supervision. We do not merely seek to give the supervisee insight; we want the supervisee to experience his/her triangling patterns and options for greater differentiation within the supervision group. Less time is spent on imparting techniques for helping the supervisee to get "unstuck" with his therapy case. Theoretically, we assume that the therapist's problem is not primarily a lack of information. Our conclusion is that he/she recreates structures in therapy with families that are isomorphic with family-of-origin contexts. These structures inhibit creative extrication from "stuckness". Suggestions of techniques are most appropriate after the triangling structure is dealt with.

While we encourage greater self-differentiation for supervisees, we believe this use of the supervision group is distinct from therapy. The focus is on a presentation of a case. Further, interactions, patterns of triangling and emotional fusion by the supervisee are discussed in terms of his/her relationship to case management and role as therapist.

Suggestions of specific techniques for getting unstuck are always appropriate. Before and after experiences of dealing with one's structure of triangling within the group, members can observe how the supervisee handles the suggestions (i.e., were the suggestions followed or dismissed). Just offering techniques for getting unstuck in therapy is not enough. The combination of techniques and group supervision is needed.

THE ROLE OF INSIGHT FROM THE FAMILY OF ORIGIN

We assume that patterns of interpersonal behavior learned in the supervisee's family of origin will be repeated with families in therapy and within the supervisory group. When something about the therapeutic or supervisory situation triggers anxiety in the supervisee, he/she will then react with the same patterns of triangulation experienced over time in the family of origin. Through the use of the genogram, the supervisory group helps the supervisee identify major patterns of family of origin fusion and triangulation. The emphasis is then on how these patterns are re-enacted in present interpersonal situations.

As an example, one common pattern of triangulation often seen in clinical trainees involves that of the interpersonal style of the over-functioner and under-functioner (Burden, 1980). The over-functioner chooses to avoid anxiety by being in charge and taking care of another. The under-functioner deals with anxiety by having another on whom he/she can depend. This pattern was identified in one supervisee who was fused in the triangulation involving her older sister, her mother and herself. Whenever she experienced her mother demanding certain behaviors from her, she would adopt a position of weakness. Her older sister would then rescue her by helping her with the required behavior and siding with her against mother. This repetitive triangular sequence would lead the supervisee to adopt an under-functioning role while her older sister maintained a position of over-responsibility. Both were coalesced against mother.

At times during therapy sessions, as well as in group supervisory sessions, this supervisee would feel confused and stressed. She would then adopt an under-functioning role which would encourage others to take care of her. In therapy sessions, it was not unusual for her to elicit support from one family member while remaining helpless with another. In group supervision, she was skilled at getting another group member to come to her rescue when the supervisor was raising her anxiety level around some issue. As this supervisee became more aware of her role in the under-functioning triangulation process within the supervisory group, she was able to initiate different behaviors which also carried over into her therapy with families.

THE ROLE OF INSIGHT FROM THE FAMILY CONSTELLATION

The use of family constellation information, early recollections and dream material as discussed by Adler (1958) and Toman (1976) enable the supervisee to grasp the specific idiosyncratic patterns of emotional triangling from his/her family of origin rather quickly. This information and the family genogram, in combination with the group experience, provide an intense impetus for differentiation.

The family constellation material is gathered from perceived sibling order characteristics (Toman, 1976) with more specific idiographic detail of patterns of emotional fusion garnered from early recollections (Adler, 1958) and dreams. Adler (1958) argues that early recollections are selected from millions of experiences because they dramatically represent the particular view of life (beliefs) which the individual uses to guide him/her through anxiety. It is expected that early patterns of learned triangulation not only are captured in these memories, but that the beliefs contained in them continue to operate in the individual's present triangling maneuvers. Dream material is assumed to reflect dramatic representations of problem-solving based on the underlying beliefs found in the early recollections. We believe that these patterns will show up in therapy and in the group supervision experience.

An example of these patterns can be seen in a supervisee who reported frequently leaving out the mother, responding more to the father and overlooking children in her therapy with families. Her posture and seating position (from videotapes) was usually directed toward the father with significantly more verbal communications directed to him. She would respond when the mother tried to talk but would soon move back to the father. When these issues were discussed during group supervision the supervisee directed most of her responses, overt and covert, toward the male supervisor and other males in the group. Female supervisees who attempted to make comments were passed over.

The supervisee had two older brothers who, it could be expected, grew up protecting her. Her early recollections contained themes of males (older brothers) entertaining her, sacrificing themselves for her (her brother got stung by bees while keeping her safe) and several recollections in which male support was conspicuously absent, but strongly desired by her. When females were supportive in her recollections their support was taken for granted by the supervisee. Often females were seen by her as competitive. Mother was described as "always there" and appeared to be taken for granted. Father was frequently absent, because of his job, and his returns home were full of excitement and specialness. In stressful situations, as dramatized by her dreams, anxiety was coped with by males supporting and rescuing her in frightening circumstances. Supportive males seemed to be present throughout her life. She contributed to their presence by trying to please them, being loyal and regularly communicating her need for their help.

It was not surprising that these patterns of triangulation and fusion would show up in this woman's therapy and supervision. Some understanding of the supervisee's interactional patterns could have been gained outside of a group supervision model. However, the group's experience of the patterns enabled greater clarity and a more profound understanding of the precursors (body cues, physical sensations, multiple communication levels) of the fusion.

A significant contribution by the supervision group was to provide an experience in which supervisor/members did not allow themselves to be put in supportive roles (i.e., triangulated). This created an intensity which pushed the supervisee to try new, more differentiated options of relating to the supervisory group members. The supervisee's opportunity to relate more assertively in the group supervision enabled her to initiate different patterns in therapy with families.

PROTOCOL FOR INTEGRATED MODEL OF SUPERVISION

During the first year of training in family therapy, supervisees take coursework in various family therapies (e.g., structural, strategic, Bowen and Milan schools). They begin a family-of-origin group their first year which includes a thorough examination of each student's genogram, family constellation, and early recollection/dream material. During the second year of training, after active family therapy practice has begun, the supervisees begin the weekly group supervision experience. At each supervisee's initial video presentation a brief summary of his/her family of origin, early recollection/dream material is presented. Then a videotape of an active case is shown. Selected portions are highlighted by the group. In these segments, the supervisee assesses how triangulating patterns were activated and managed. Also discussed are bodily cues and potential options for changing patterns of response in future sessions. Group interaction becomes the on-going focus with special attention given to how triangulating is activated in the group.

CONCLUSION

This model of family therapy supervision should be viewed first as an attempt to develop an approach to supervision that is isomorphic with the therapy practiced by the supervisee. The particular content of this model represents the authors' theoretical biases and, as such, reflects only an example of how models of supervision in family therapy can be developed. Whatever the particular content of one's supervision, clarity and direction will be enhanced if one's supervisory approach is consistent with the family therapy treatment taught and practiced in the training model.

REFERENCES

Adler, A. (1958). *What life should mean to you.* Capricorn Books.
Ard, D. (1973). Providing clinical supervision for marriage counselors: A model for Supervisor and Supervisee. *Family Coordinator,* 22: 91-98.
Berger, M. and Dammann, C. (1982). Live supervision as context, treatment and training. *Family Process,* 21, 337-344.
Bowen, M. (1978). *Family therapy in clinical practice.* New York: Jason Aronson.
Burden, S. (1980). Tracking over-responsibility in a family system. *The Family,* 8, 42-45.
Cormier, L. and Bernard, J. (1982). Ethical and legal responsibilities of clinical supervisors. *Personnel and Guidance Journal,* 60(8), 486-490.
Fisher, B. and Keele, R. (1981). The kingdom of Guru: A parable of supervision. *Family Therapy,* 8(2), 129-134.
Hart, G. (1982). *The process of clinical supervision.* Baltimore, Maryland, University Park Press.
Keller, J.F. and Protinsky, H. (1984). A self-management model for supervision. *Journal of Marital and Family Therapy.* 109(3), 281-288.
Liddle, H. and Halpin, R. (1978). Family therapy training and supervision literature: A comparative review. *Journal of Marriage and Family Counseling,* 4, 77-98.
Montalvo, B. (1973). Aspects of live supervision. *Family Process,* 12, 343-359.
Protinsky, H. and Keller, J.F. (1984). Supervision of marriage and family therapy: A family of origin approach. *The Clinical Supervisor,* 2(2), 75-80.
Toman, W. (1976). *Family constellation.* New York: Springer.

Toward Cognitive-Behavioral Integration in Training Systems Therapists: An Interactive Approach to Training in Generic Systems Thinking

Bunny S. Duhl

ABSTRACT. This paper describes the integrative approach to training in systems thinking developed at the Boston Family Institute. Specifically, an experiential-cognitive training model is described in terms of Piagetian theory, learning styles, metaphor, and exercises which bridge right- and left-brain processes. This model is intended to connect trainees' personal experiences with systems theory and therapeutic skills.

"Intelligence thus begins neither with knowledge of the self nor of things as such, but with knowledge of their interaction, and it is by orienting itself simultaneously toward the two poles of that interaction that intelligence organizes the world by organizing itself."
(Piaget, in Gruber & Voneche, 1977, p. 275).

To think systemically means *to see how all component parts FIT in dynamic interaction with each other,* or more simply, how people fit together in patterned interactions. In the 1960s, many old ways of teaching did not seem to work to help trainees grasp both the sense of interpersonal interconnection (relationships), AND ways of working with those interconnections (interventions which influence changes in relationships). At this time, material concerning WHAT comprised family system interconnections, that is, the betweenness of family members, and HOW to interact with families in ways that could help them alter their relationships, was very much in the process of being discovered and invented, as were ways to teach these new discoveries. Teaching family systems therapy then involved, and still involves, providing the context for learning *about* how people interconnect (cognitive learning) as well as providing an opportu-

---

Bunny S. Duhl, Ed.D., is Co-Director of the Boston Family Institute. She may be reached at 55 Williston Road, Brookline, MA 02146.

nity to learn how family members behave, and how therapists, new trainees, perform as interveners (behavioral learning).

When the Boston Family Institute (BFI) was started in 1969 by people from the mental health field,[1] several questions were uppermost in the minds of the trainers, questions which have remained constant over the years: 1) How do people learn? 2) What are families and other living systems? 3) How can the process of teaching fit the process of learning? and 4) How can the content and the process by which people learn be congruent with each other and the process of therapy?

These are complex questions to which answers did not appear immediately, but evolved over 15 years and continue to evolve today. The trainers at BFI, through active and conscious experimentation, arrived at a new *interactive* mode of training, an experiential/cognitive model in which the "theory-in-use" is congruent with the "theory as espoused" (Argyris and Schon, 1974; Schon, 1975), where processes of teaching are congruent with processes of learning, and where teaching/learning is congruent with the tasks and contexts of therapy.

Over the years, adult trainees have reported themselves as "more integrated" that is, feeling centered inside themselves as persons and as therapists, having an awareness of their own human experience but still open to continued learning, able to be both excited and comfortable, and at the same time expand their behavioral range as therapists. These are unusual statements and invited my curiosity.

An exploration of this way of teaching viewed through the theoretical lenses of certain learning theorists has helped me to make sense of the phenomena trainees describe. The puzzle I focused on relates to this expressed sense of centered openness that I now call cognitive/behavioral integration. Piaget, Bruner, Gordon and a cadre of brain/mind researchers are of particular significance in lending coherence to this integration.

This paper explores several constructs which shed light on the *fit* of teaching/learning processes at BFI which seem to promote this integration in the trainees. I hope that others may find these constructs useful in their training programs. The BFI experiential/cognitive model of training:

a. Taps into and exercises all four basic stages of cognition described by Piaget (1952), leading to cognitive/behavioral awareness and flexibility;

b. Employs the connective learning processes of metaphor described by Gordon (1961), allowing for reciprocal and reversible flow be-

---

[1]Particularly responsible for this approach were the founders of BFI, David Kanter, Ph.D., and Frederick J. Duhl, M.D. The author and Jeremy Cobb, M.A., among others, became instrumental in continuing to shape this approach during its early years.

tween image and idea, between construct and behavior; between behavior, image and idea;
  c. Provides ''exercise'' for the integration of right and left brain types
     of learning described by Ornstein (1972), Bogen (1968), Deikman
     (1968), Duhl & Duhl (1981), and others, promoting a wide range of
     avenues for connection of experience and theory;
  d. Provides room for exploration of different types of learning styles
     (Duhl & Duhl, 1975), promoting greater fit of teaching/learning
     processes as well as promoting each trainee to be in charge of
     his/her learning;
  e. ''Honors each student'' (Gordon, 1977) by drawing on his/her own
     knowledge and experience, fostering centeredness and confidence;
  f. Provides for the integration of theory and the development of con-
     gruence.
  g. Honors the ''Having of wonderful ideas'' (Duckworth, 1972),
     which I would maintain ''is the essense of intellectual development''
     for adults as well as children.

At this point, let me begin to fill in the picture with the theoretical
framework taught at BFI.

THE CONTENT: A VERY BRIEF SKETCH OF GENERAL
SYSTEMS THEORY AND FAMILY SYSTEMS

The Boston Family Institute program trains people to work with families, in whole or in parts, by developing the map, or metaphor, of family
systems, inside each trainee's mind. This *generic systems theory,* the
foundation of all training at the Boston Family Institute, is based on von
Bertalanffy's general systems theory which he first applied to cell biology, and subsequently extended with others to people and to all living systems (Gray, Duhl, & Rizzo, 1969; von Bertalanffy, 1969, Duhl & Duhl,
1981; Duhl, 1983).
In systems theory, the family is seen as a continuously developing
system, with subsystem patterns that tend to stay in balance and in dynamic tension with each other. The process of stabilizing and accommodating changes into the total family system is the work of the family. The
same theory applies to all levels of living systems such as to individuals
and their physiological systems as well as to the community outside the
family.
Each person embodies entire patterns learned, mostly out of awareness, in his/her family of origin, and pre-marriage environments and
experience. Each person's way of doing things, looking at the world, perceiving and giving meaning to behaviors and events, are contextually re-

lated. Bruner calls this type of learning "incidental learning" or "past history" (Bruner, 1973).

In our changing multi-cultural society, the subsystem of the married couple is made up of the mix and mosaic of previously learned patterns of each individual, which form a new arrangement of patterns as the couple lives together over time. The couple's patterned interactions (system) then help shape the new arrivals, the children, in combination with each child's biologically inherited predispositions. As in all systems, the style, timing and context of the new arrival (the child) impacts *on* the parents as much as the parents impact *on* the child. For instance, the loss of a loved one by a parent prior to the birth of a child is a *system former* (Gray, 1976) and influences how that new child will be received into the family. If we apply Piaget's terms to reciprocal influences in families, each family member is *assimilating* and *accommodating* to the others.

INTERPERSONAL ISSUES IN FAMILIES

The basic interpersonal issues within families parallel those of individuals throughout life. They are issues, in Piaget's terms, of assimilation, accommodation and equilibration. According to Piaget (in Gruber & Voneche, 1977),

> . . . Assimilation is conservative and tends to subordinate the environment to the organism as it is, whereas accommodation is the source of changes and bends the organism to the successive constraints of the environment...Assimilation and accommodation are therefore the two poles of an interaction between the organism and the environment. (p. 274)

These interpersonal issues in families revolve around different individuals' ways of being, perceiving, and acting. Messages and meanings given to the interactions between individuals denote their "relationship" and create their larger subsystem pattern.

We often speak of relationships and systems as if they were concrete *things*. Just as a relationship does not have physical properties, but is an experience *between* persons or things, so is a living system not physically real. "System" is but a metaphor for *patterns* of actions and relationships of component parts, which interact simultaneously as well as over time, and in doing so, elude linear description. What we call human systems then, which have an intangible psychological reality, are "wholes" of relationships which we can grasp through metaphor. These intangible metaphors of betweenness are what systems therapists attempts to change.

HOW WE LOOK AT FAMILIES AND CHANGE

The premise at BFI is that *one cannot change a relationship between people unless some behaviors, patterns, ways of thinking, acting, in individual people change.* Thus, in working with families, we note the family's life cycle stage, as well as each family's place within a multigenerational context. We look at the family system's cultural, ethnic, economic and social mix and "place" within larger systems. We also explore where each person (i.e., individual subsystem) is in his/her life cycle, the general cognitive stage and learning style of each member, health history, and the special incidents of importance to each family member. With this information in mind, we look at the automatic patterned interactions by which people live, some of which keep people locked into unrewarding and maladaptive patterns. We explore the strengths, problems, tasks, and skills needed at this time in life. We especially search out the capacity of the system and the individuals for novelty, change, and adaptation. Our goal is to enhance the functional autonomy of each individual while each remains in viable connection with others.

In this respect, the Boston Family Institute's model is primarily a cognitive and contextual learning model rather than a sickness/cure medical model. Interventions are based on not one specific set of techniques, but arise from an assessment of which types of intervention best *fit* each family system, its context, the presenting problem, as well as each member's role, needs, information processing style, stage and mode.

It is a complicated task to think systemically in ways that do not lose touch with each individual. The individual lends shape to the larger system, just as the larger system lends shape to each individual's possibility for movement and change.

PROCESS AS CONTENT: SOME THOUGHTS ABOUT LEARNING STYLES, STAGES AND MODES

Piaget (Ginsburg & Opper, 1969; Piaget, 1952; Piaget & Inhelder, 1969; Flavell, 1963, 1977) and his colleagues have postulated and established to their satisfaction that there are set sequences in learning or cognitive stages in all "normal" human beings. They further postulate that while these stages always follow the same sequence, they do not always develop in a set time. In addition, the structures in each stage do not necessarily develop equivalently, "across the board" or at a uniform rate within one person in different areas of development. *While this material is important to keep in mind when working with families, it is equally important to consider when training adults.*

Similarly, although it is postulated that people have the maturational and developmental capacity to reach the formal operational stage by adolescence, not all do so by that time or perhaps, ever. In addition, an implication can be drawn from Piaget's work that if one has reached the formal operational stage in one arena, he or she will be able to reason abstractly in another. In practice, we have found that this is not so. A brilliant chemist does not necessarily impose the same type of ability in his/her personal relationships as he/she does in his/her chemical experiments. When people come into training, they too represent a diversity of levels of abilities to think both concretely and abstractly about human begins in groups we call systems. Similarly, they differ in how they take in and process information, give it meaning and store it (Duhl & Duhl, 1975).

THE BACKGROUND FOR THE PROCESS OF LEARNING

Differentiating Cognitive Stages From Styles. It is important also to make a distinction between the level or stage of one's cognitive development and the style of functioning within that level or stage. Issues of different infant styles have been described by Thomas and Chess (1977) and others, as "temperamental differences." Similarly, temperament can be applied and enlarged upon in the concept of learning styles. Certain aspects of learning style tend to stay the same from childhood into adult life. Indigenous characteristics are enhanced or thwarted by the contexts in which people live, grow and learn from infancy through adulthood. Few contexts enhance cognitive/behavioral integration.

Foxes and Hedgehogs. Consider Aristotle's analogy of the fox and the hedgehog as representing two polarities of styles of thinking and being.

In catching a chicken, the fox jumps all over the field, keeps an eye on his prey, hides behind the tall grass, and confuses the chicken by racing in a circle. Finally, he pounces, getting the chicken. The hedgehog also gets the chicken, moving slowly, deliberately, and quietly in a straight line. Their styles are obviously very different. One is analogic, the other digital (Duhl & Duhl, 1975).

The analogic fox thinks associatively, making internal leaps across categories when making connections (paralleling what brain researchers [Ornstein, 1972] have labeled "right-brain" thinking). The digital hedgehog thinks in a step-by-step fashion, down one path at a time, rarely jumping across categories. Rather than move to another path, the hedgehog must either back up and start anew, or take a well-marked bridge from one path to the next. Speed is not an issue, for some hedgehogs can move very fast down each path. (This linear style may be linked to the "left-brain" thinking described by Bogen and others.) When you put foxes and hedgehogs together without a mediator or process of bridging, then conflict arises with put down, irritation, annoyance, blame and other offensive/defensive maneuvers.

Sensory Modes and Channels in Learning or Information Processing. Other aspects of learning style relate to predominant sensory intake channels and sequences of information processing. There are those who must see something done before they can integrate, understand it, and begin to do it. Written instructions for them do not convey the imagistic gestalts by which their comprehension takes place. Such people often think in images and struggle to find the language to describe these images.

There are those who order their information primarily through auditory channels and need to hear first what is expected and how to do it, before they can proceed. These people use words to create a thought as well as to order a sequence in their mind.

And there are those who jump in and physically tackle a task with no previous information, and then step back and seek out a visual or auditory cue before proceeding. These people often read instructions or consult an expert *after* exploring a matter, with specific questions provoked by their hands-on exploration.

What This Means for Training. We have found, through years of experience, that each person's style varies along three dimensions of information processing: social, academic, and physical. We have also found that one dimension often is independent of another.

It is our postulation that *both* the Piagetian stage or level of cognitive development and the learning style within that stage or level, are important factors in each individual's ability to connect with others, fit comfortably in families and continue to learn as adults. Rarely, however, is there the opportunity for individuals to explore their own learning styles in order to enhance their own learning potential and integration, as well as to understand systemically how stage and style are factors of FIT in families and other systems. No trainee or workshop participant in our 15 year experience had ever been asked prior to his/her BFI experience to explore how he/she processed information in different arenas, nor how that style fit with others in his/her family system and other contexts.

Other factors influencing how individuals process information, interact, and participate in close relationships include how people use time, space and energy (Kantor & Lehr, 1975) the periodicity in internal body rhythms and energy (Luce, 1971), and other biological entities at both the cellular and organ levels. In addition, each person gives meaning to these factors in themselves and in others, and they become important in terms of relationship development and maintenance. Rarely are they distilled out as biological factors with origins devoid of motive.

Other "Modes" of Thinking: Right Brain, Left Brain and Piaget. In the past decade or so, much attention has been paid to different learning or thinking styles, or modes, attributed to the right and left hemispheres of the brain (see Ornstein, 1972; Gazzaniga, 1967; Deikman, 1971; de Bono, 1970; Bogen, 1969;). Basically, the myths (dating back to the I

Ching), concepts, theories and research postulate that the right side of the brain is responsible for nonlinear thinking, imagery, spatial relationships, simultaneity, and gestalts, while the left side is responsible for linear, verbal, propositional logical thought. Activating the usually ignored right brain is very important in training people in systems thinking, since by their very nature, considering human systems involves spatial relationships, gestalts, and imagery.

Also, different kinds of problem-solving appears to involve different aspects of brain activity, as found in brain wave research (Deikman, 1971). Similarly, different modes of teaching call on and use different sides of the brain (Bruner, 1976; Buzan, 1976; Konicek, 1976; de Bono, 1970).

Interestingly enough, while Piaget has generally been seen as the explorer of left brain functions, his paper on "The Role of Imitation in the Development of Representational Thought", alludes to different aspects of thought that seem to fit these right and left brain categories:

> . . . Representational thought exhibits a *"figural"* nature, i.e., it tends to provide an image that more or less conforms to represented realities, i.e., configurations . . . Representation may also involve transformations as such and deal more with operations and constructions than with copying . . . it would even seem that the totality of cognitive functions derives from such a dichotomy. (Piaget, in Gruber and Voneche, 1977, p. 512) [Italics mine]

Piaget also felt that "the figural aspect and the operative aspect of representational thought are basically complementary" (p. 514). As such, Piaget may be underscoring the importance of developing both sides of the brain.

Piaget (Gruber and Voneche, 1977) speaks of thought as internalized action, and states that body action is at the base of all thought. Moreover, he seems to indicate that different types of body actions lead to different modes of thought. This may be true for adults as well as young children.

THE RELATIONSHIPS OF STYLE, STAGES, AND MODES TO TRAINING

These various ways of looking at how the brain/mind works all underlie how people process information, their cognitive stages, and learning styles. In the training program at the Boston Family Institute, *in addition to traditional reading and paper writing,* we design a myriad of exercises that tap into different learning styles, stages and modes (behavioral learning) and debrief them (cognitive learning) in ways that people may learn constructs from their own experience. Trainees later interview (behavioral learning) a) each other in role played families, b) non-care-seeking families in front of peers, and finally c) care-seeking families. All of these interviews are reviewed and debriefed (cognitive learning) with others.

Metaphor Ties It All Together

In a remarkable article by Jimenez (1976), entitled *Piaget and Synectics,* Jimenez takes Piaget's assimilation and accommodation processes and ties them together with W.J.J. Gordon's (1961) ideas of creative problem-solving through the use of analogy and metaphor.

According to Jimenez, Gordon states that "the mind has two basic jobs to perform. One is to 'Make the Strange Familiar,'[2] that is, to incorporate new facts, events, experience, etc., into the frameworks already established by previously appropriated facts, events, experiences, etc." This process of *connection-making* Gordon (1961) calls *learning,* and is the process of assimilation which occurs in play.

According to Jimenez' (1976) account of Gordon, "The other process of intelligence is the opposite. It is to 'Make the Familiar Strange' that is, to free something already known from the stereotypes we have put into it . . . to alter one's angle of vision to meet new realities." This is a process that Gordon calls *innovation* or *connection-breaking* and Piaget calls accommodation, which is accomplished by imitation. "Here, the child adapts himself to what he sees, and tries to understand it by imitating it, getting the feel of it from inside . . . " (Jimenez, 1976).

According to Jimenez (1976), then, "Children's play is a form of 'Making the Strange Familiar', or of simply keeping everything as familiar as possible," of reducing the world to the child. "Children's imitation is a form of 'Making the Familiar Strange', of exploring the unknown," which through "the work of metaphor expands the world to the child . . . Metaphor is the simple device by which the mind, both child and adult, accomplishes its twin prodigies."

Metaphor, in Greek, means "carrying from one place to another." In the BFI training program, we design exercises as experiential metaphors and analogies to real life situations. These exercises involve both play and imitation (Duhl, 1983), which make the Strange Familiar and the Familiar Strange. Each exercise and debriefing session carries experiences and ideas from one place to another.

SOME OVERVIEWS OF TRAINING

Training involves the broadening of the maps or sets by which the therapist observes and acts as well as broadening the therapist's skills. The

---

[2]I will capitalize Strange and Familiar as Gordon does, for emphasis of the concept.

goal of training is to help the therapist develop a wide range of maps and behaviors that help families and other human systems change their mental sets and behaviors. Mental sets change when missing information is filled in (Making the Strange Familiar), and when reality is challenged and re-framed (Making the Familiar Strange).

At BFI we choose people for training who have some observable sense of empathy and are able to report and make sense for themselves of what they have just experienced. We are most concerned with how applicants look at the interactions between people, and we scan for a developing sense of system and metaphor in potential trainees.

We believe it is important to study the non-care-seeking family before we study how to influence the family in distress. It is important for people to recognize what is ordinary and usual so they may know the full contin-uum towards jeopardy (Duhl & Duhl, 1981). Thus, a solid year is spent in rearranging the maps of the mind before trainees are expected to be of service to families in need. During this year, in addition to an experien-tially based seminar in systems thinking, trainees explore theory in other more didactic seminars.

Since we cannot have many families study day in and day out at BFI, and since every trainee is a representative of at least one family system we teach family systems by using the raw data of trainees' lives and families as samples. Through analogy and metaphor, in action as well as words, each learns about the theory and reality of family systems.

Discovering the "Set"

To train people to be change agents, on line, with families, in a setting where the only tool is oneself, means also to train people to know what "set" or representative systems they already carry in their minds. If peo-ple do not know what their own "set" is, they will impose it blindly on whatever new situation is in front of them.

Certain already coded "data" (i.e., a trainee's past experiences) are equivalent to a closed system, in that they are out of awareness and not available. At BFI we have felt it is necessary to make that which is taken for granted, overt. We do this through metaphor. We design exercises which draw forth what trainees have already encoded concerning family systems by tapping into their own past history. In this sense, we are "Making the Familiar Strange," in Gordon's terms. Metaphor "evokes the preconscious, and watches it work" (Gordon, 1961).

Thus, during that first year, trainees engage in exercises that tap into family rules, stories, roles, contexts, learning styles, decision-making processes, rituals, vulnerabilities, defenses, conflict styles, boundary be-havior, ethnic and contextual history, core images, networks, myths, and much more. Over time, the epistemic map emerges, and is already being changed through exposure to the maps of others.

When the Familiar is made strange over and over again, trainees learn to learn options. They learn to learn that how one looks and intervenes and labels depends on where one stands, his/her "set" or "professional deformation." Trainees become aware of the relative "truth" in any belief system, and the importance of context in shaping human beings.

We already know, in addition to many different "sets" entering a training program that there will be many different samples of learning styles and levels of cognitive development. For instance, we have found that those people who are perhaps most advanced in their formal operational processes are often those who are most out of touch with their own experiences and with other people. They are often good strategy planners, but very poor on-line therapists, since they often do not know how to personally enact the myriad steps of connection and of "getting to here from there" with the family members.

Similarly, we often find that people who are most in touch with their own and others' feelings may not have the vaguest idea what strategy is needed to help a family from disabling or "stuck" patterns to enabling ones.

The trainers, then, design exercises (metaphors) to capture a concept, which also involves learning through sensorimotor activity, and activities that incorporate preoperational, concrete operational and formal operational structures. We try to design for active and receptive modes, for foxes and hedgehogs, for see-ers, and do-ers. We do much of this through metaphor.

When we then ask in debriefing, "What did you learn? And with what else does that connect?" we are exercising each trainee's capacity for cognitive integration of experientially derived data.

By using interactive metaphors in teaching we are making the Familiar Strange. This innovative process of breaking connections, toward new facts and feelings to be learned (Gordon & Poze, 1977) not only opens the "set," but provides for "diversity of training" (Bruner, 1973).

To sum up then, we take the "personal data" of people's lives—their experiences and sets—as well as published "outside data," and transform it by setting up experiential metaphoric exercises which invite generalizations, concepts and theories. We do this in such a way that each exercise simultaneously is available to different learning styles and cognitive stages.

The Challenge of a Curriculum

Over the course of the past fifteen years, an integrated curriculum has been developed at BFI. The goals, hypotheses, assumptions, and exercises for each seminar are designed specifically for each session and copies of the daily curriculum are given to trainees at the end of each session. This process ensures a structure to the spontaneity of the teaching, makes us accountable to ourselves as well as our trainees, keeps our creative and growing edge sharp with the challenge of finding yet another way to get an old concept across, and gives us and trainees a weekly record of where we have been on the way to where we are going.

From the Theory to the Process

One of the first ways in which we "Make the Familiar Strange" is to use the symbolic language of pantomine or nonverbal interactions, by which we can represent total intrapsychic or interactional situations. For example, a memory is an image, like a dream. One can ask people to use themselves and others to represent the memory-dream in space. After all, that is what theatre is all about—a playwrights' image of people in relationships represented in space (Duhl, 1983). In the sense that we are externalizing in spatial metaphor people's words or unspoken images and thoughts, we are "Making the Familiar Strange." In so doing, people can step back, take a look and make new connections and new learnings. In this process, in Piagetian terms, we are taking that which has been assimilated and externalizing it through the use of verbal and spatial metaphors so that a new accommodation takes place.

Looking at one well-known exercise in a day's curriculum may help the reader understand the theory-in-use.

An Exercise in Analysis of an Exercise

Topic: The use of the spatial metaphor of Sculpture. The goal of the exercise is to explore emotional closeness and distance in a trainee's own family or one in treatment. Using what is the now well-known process of sculpture (Duhl, Kantor, Duhl, 1973; Duhl, B., 1983) we ask a trainee to choose others in the seminar to represent family members (with the trainee playing him/herself), and place them so that the distance between persons would represent emotional closeness, not only to the trainee, but also to each other family member. We then ask him/her to give each "family member" a gesture or series of gestures that represented the attitudes of that person to other "family members." Since family systems take place in real time and space, we ask the trainee to put this scene into a dance-like motion, indicating who moves closer to whom, away from whom, and what happens.

All of the above, once explained by the trainee is enacted without words perhaps several times—at normal speed, quite fast, and in slow motion, so that the sense of pattern is heightened as well as the individual actions taken. At the end of this process, we ask each of the players as well as observers for a verbal metaphor that represents the process in the family system.

We then debrief. Most often, we ask each player, "How did it feel to be who you were in this role? What did you learn about yourself in this role? About yourself in relation to others? What did you learn about the whole system?" In the process of relating his/her new awareness, each player is giving information to the trainee and others of his/her reactions, interpretations, and meanings based on his/her sensorimotor activities, as well as on his "postural" or proprioceptive system. Each person is also learning about him/herself.

What has happened? Let us look at this exercise both in terms of theoretical constructs and in terms of behavioral/cognitive integration.

The trainee has to conjure up past images of his/her family members in interactions with each other. The trainee must then make a leap from image-memories, which could be approximated by having others "imitate" these memories, to an abstraction involving emotions and space. The trainee is constantly *assimilating* and taking in what is in his environment and memories, and is *accommodating* those memories to the present environment by placing people in space. As the trainee thinks of distance between people as representing emotional distance, he/she is basically accommodating, making the Familiar Strange.

As each player gives his/her feedback, the trainee or "sculptor" assimilates a *multicentric view* —the same experience from several different yet simultaneous perceptions. The resultant effect of this process on the trainee aids him/her in *decentering,* through the awareness that there is no one perception, no one correct view, of a total system process. In Gordon's terms, we have made the Familiar egocentric view very Strange indeed.

Verbal Metaphors

When we ask all present to think of a metaphor that captures the family's systemic interaction, we are very much in Gordon's (1961) realm. We are asking them to make a Direct Analogy (e.g., this family is like a "merry-go-round," "a spider's web," a "non-stop train"). By the use of such imagery, Gordon postulates that people can remove themselves to a different vantage point, and see something more clearly. In so doing, and in making associative leaps, the "leaper" is making his/her own connections, and in the process, learning, integrating. The metaphor then becomes the glue of connection, and of internalization, of joining the assimilating and accommodation processes. Our experience has been that trainees tend to remember with vividness each other's sculptures and metaphors. In addition, such metaphors allow them to "hold" the family system in mind in ways that later connect with theoretical descriptions of family systems. (Such theoretical descriptions are but a different kind of metaphor and are no more or less "real" than those of the trainees.)

From Specifics to Generalizations

After we have "sculpted" and debriefed several vignettes of trainees' families during a seminar, we ask for generalizations about the process, about families, about learnings derived from the experience. These generalizations tend to range from observations (paralleling Piaget's preoperational and concrete operational stages) to levels of generalization that have to do, for instance, with "emotional field forces," "entropy," "deviation amplification" (formal operational stage). During one such exercise, trainees may be taken through parallels to all four Piagetian stages of development.

During debriefing, we validate the new discoveries, the new "wonderful ideas," the "aha's" that trainees come up with in the course of a sculpture, all of which are the buds of new integration and theory. Each owns the discovery process, which each then begins to weave into theory from the inside out (Duhl, 1983).

We ask trainees to write each week in their journals their own associations about what has seemed important, what they have learned. Periodically, we ask for an integration of their learnings through written papers, diagrams, and other modes of presentation. We respect each trainee's learning style by requesting that each be competent in the mode that fits each the best, yet also ask for left-brain, verbal, linear integration of nonlinear right-brain material.

Other Exercises Analyzed: Underscoring Cognitive Stages

Over the years, while exploring other content and/or developing therapy skills, we have developed a number of exercises or procedures which zero in more on one cognitive stage parallel than another. Some samples follow.

1) *The Sensorimotor Level:*
Exercise. Pick a partner and plan to play "follow the leader." First leader: Walk around the room in your normal gait. Follower, follow, in body posture and rhythm. Leader: Then imagine yourself feeling very joyful. Walk in that way, follower following. Leader: now imagine yourself feeling and walk in that body posture and rhythm. Switch roles. Repeat sequence. Debrief.

In this exercise, we are asking trainees to expand their sense of empathy with others. In this, we have them "go back to basics" in showing and doing with their bodies in action, as they did in Follow the Leader as children, and to walk in each other's shoes. Action in space more closely approximates another's direct experience than words. When one walks in another's rhythm and gait, one approximates another's way of being in body, feelings, meanings, and style. In addition, the trainee adds to his/her own multicentricity, by incorporating awareness of other styles of being. Such exercises do expand the sense of empathy. Each "follower" *discovers* from the inside out during such approximations, how another possibly feels. This nonverbal language quickly augments verbal language with families.

With other such nonverbal exercises, trainees learn to stop and ask for pantomine meanings of *any* terms/words about which there is disagreement. In that way, idiosyncratic meanings are clarified for their differences and nuances (Duhl, 1983). Trainees are expected to ask family members to do the same thing, since meanings of relationship is what conflict is about.

2) *The Pre-operational Stage:*
Exercise. A group of 3-5 trainees works out a pantomime representing one person's learning style sequence, with the rest of the group as audience. Debriefing begins with: What did you *see?* asked of the observers.

As trainees begin to answer with interpretations, as they invariably do, we label them interpretations, and ask again and again—"What did you *see?*" until the observers describe sequences of actions observed, devoid of interpretive meaning. We then ask, "What meaning do you attribute to what you saw?" Then we ask the actors to acknowledge those who guessed their meanings correctly, and to explain whatever was misread. Those who enacted the sequence also learn how precisely or imprecisely they have transmitted their messages.

In this exercise we are developing trainees observational skills of sequences and process while interrupting the automatic precoded meanings each brings into the room. It is exceedingly hard not to give meaning—to interrupt the schemata we have formed and take for granted. In this type of exercise, the formerly Familiar is made Strange and new. Egocentric meanings often do not apply. In this process, trainees learn to ask questions to check out their assumptions. Being able to track sequences without interpreting is essential for a therapist, in order to see the patterns, be able to enquire and appreciate what sequences and dialogues mean to the people having them, and in order to help people *see* and *hear* each other.

3) *The Concrete Operational Stage and Decentration:*
Exercise. Several trainees are asked to role play a family seen in

therapy with the trainee-therapists taking two significant family roles. Two other trainees are asked to interview the family. The remainder are "observer/supervisors." Trainees debrief this exercise in a wide variety of ways, including asking the original therapists what they learned from their role-played parts. Observers are asked how it felt to watch this interview and supervise.

In training therapists, we are training people in role taking in the Piagetian sense—that ability to be empathic with others. By employing many kinds of role taking and role enactment we are making the Strange Familiar, in Gordon's terms, and again setting up a context for decentration in Piaget's terms. When trainees roleplay the people they are treating, they gain new awareness of interpersonal dynamics and discover new ways of reaching formerly "unreachable" clients. When trainees roleplay supervisors, they must see/comprehend and be responsible for the whole larger system, the therapist-family system.

Decentration, a critical capacity for systems therapists to have, is a process which involves both assimilation and accommodation, making the Strange Familiar and the Familiar Strange. It involves the coordination of separate points of views, separate realities.

When trainees are put in as many skins as possible, they move flexibly between Strange and Familiar. For what we aspire to is that decentered position for therapists in which the Familiar is Strange enough not to be taken for granted and the Strange is Familiar enough not to be frightening and unmasterable.

4) *The Formal Operational Level:*

Exercise. In our theory lab, trainees are asked to read, for example, Bowen's theory on triangles and triangulation in families (Anonymous, 1972). In this course, they are asked to keep a journal which tracks their own associations, their own "wonderful ideas" while they are reading Bowen. In the seminar, we first discuss their own associations. Then we ask them to map their own family system in terms of Bowen's theory—in triangles. In this, we are asking, does his theory fit anything you know? Then we will ask them to put all personal associations and reflections aside, and look at Bowen's theory and track it for its internal logic. Does it hold? Is anything left out? Does each premise follow from each previous premise? What are the inherent premises or assumptions that this theory is based upon? And so on.

A good part of such a process involves intellectual, digital learning. However, we also make the Strange Familiar by providing and promoting trainee's own connective ("right brain") processes as they try out a Strange new idea from their readings with their knowledge of their own Familiar families. These are assimilatory processes. At the point at which we put the familiar aside, and look at the theory itself (now made familiar), trainees are not struggling with its content any longer, or struggling with agreement or disagreement. They are free to look at it in a depersonalized way. This is an accommodation process, in that it is making the Familiar Strange. Trainees are being asked to expand and use their "left-brain" logical processes, and push themselves beyond the information given (Bruner, 1973).

When we ask them to track a theory's internal logic, and to derive the implications of a theory, we are calling on the formal operational ("left brain") structures of each trainee. They accomplish this easily because we have taken them "up the ladder" from the personal and known, validating their ideas along the way, to the impersonal new material, which has become somewhat known in the process. By the time we are discussing, for instance, triangulation, and undifferentiated ego mass, those concepts are already connected to some experience in each trainee's life. Though these concepts and theories are abstractions, they do not float unattached to experience. Consequently, trainees begin to look for the real life examples which theories postulate or describe, as well as create their own theories from multiple real life examples.

SUMMARY

In this paper, I have attempted to link theoretical constructs of several learning theorists and brain researchers to the interactive way of teaching generic systems thinking developed at the Boston Family Institute. These constructs seem to illuminate that sense of cognitive/behavioral integration that trainees describe, in which they feel more autonomous and centered in themselves, as therapists, while also open to new ideas and new learning. This experiential/cognitive approach to training is felt to enhance that integration in the trainee by exercising parallels to all four stages of Piagetian development, by exploring each trainee's learning style, drawing material from trainee's own lives in addition to didactic material, by validating trainees' new ideas, by creating a multimodal learning environment, by designing experiences through the use of many types of analogues, metaphors, and debriefing processes thus constantly exercising right and left brain functions. This experiential/cognitive model of teaching/learning operates, then, in the service of connecting trainees' personal experience with systems theory and with therapeutic behaviors.

REFERENCES

Anonymous. (1972). Toward the differentiation of a self in one's own family. In J. L. Framo (Ed.), *Family interaction: A dialogue between family researchers and family therapist.* New York: Springer Publishing Co.

Argyris, C., & Schon, D. (1974). *Theory in practice: Increasing professional effectiveness.* San Francisco: Jossey-Bass.

Bogen, J.E. (1968). The other side of the brain: An appositional mind. In R.E. Ornstein (Ed.), *The nature of human consciousness* (pp. 101-125). San Francisco: W. H. Freeman and Co. Report *Bulletin of the Los Angeles Neurological Societies, 34,* No. 3 (July, 1969), 135-162.

Bruner, J. S. (1973). *Beyond the information given,* In J. M. Anglin (Ed.). New York: W. W. Norton and Co.

Buzan, T. (1976). *Use both sides of your brain.* New York: Dutton.

deBono, E. (1970). *Lateral thinking.* New York: Harper Colophon Books.

Deikman, A. M. (1968). Biomodal consciousness. In R. E. Ornstein (Ed.), *The nature of human consciousness.* San Francisco: W. H. Freeman and Co.

Duckworth, E. (1972). The having of wonderful ideas. *Harvard Educational Review, 42,* 217-231.

Duhl, B. S. (1983). *From the inside out and other metaphors.* New York: Brunner/Mazel.

Duhl, B. S., & Duhl, F. J. (1975). *Cognitive styles and marital process.* Paper presented at the annual meeting of the American Psychiatric Association, Anaheim, CA.

Duhl, B. S., & Duhl, F. J. (1981). Integrative family therapy. In A. Gurman & D. Kniskern (Eds.), *The handbook of family therapy.* New York: Brunner/Mazel.

Duhl, F. J., Kantor, D., & Duhl, B. S. (1973). Learning, space and action in family therapy: A primer of sculpture. In D. Bloch (Ed.), *Techniques of family psychotherapy.* New York: Grune and Stratton. Report *Seminars in Psychiatry, 5*(2), (May 1973).

Flavell, J. H. (1963). *The developmental psychology of Jean Piaget.* Princeton: Van Nostrrand Co.

Flavell, J. H. (1977). *Cognitive development.* Englewood Cliffs: Prentice-Hall.

Gazzaniga, M. S. (1968). The split brain in man. In R. E. Ornstein (Ed.), *The nature of human consciousness* (pp. 24-29). San Francisco: W. H. Freeman and Co.

Ginsburg, H., & Opper, S. (1969). *Piaget's theory of intellectual development.* Englewood Cliffs: Prentice-Hall.

Gordon, W. J. J. (1961). *Synectics: The development of creative capacity.* New York: Harper and Row.

Gordon, W. J. J. (1977, April). Connection making is university. *Curriculum Product Review.*

Gordon, W. J. J., & Poze, T. (1977, February). Toward understanding "the moment of inspiration." Presented at Creativity Symposium, American Association for the Advancement of Science.

Gray, W. (1976). The system precursor: System forming approach in General Systems Theory. Presented at VIth World Congress in Social Psychiatry, Opatija, Yugoslavia.

Gray, W., Duhl, F. J., & Rizzo, N. D. (Eds.). (1969). *General systems theory and psychiatry.* Boston: Little Brown.

Gruber, H. E., & Voneche, J. J. (Eds.). (1977). *The essential Piaget.* New York: Basic Books.

Jimenez, J. (1976). Piaget and synectics. In C. Mogdil & S. Mogdil (Eds.), *Piagetian Research Abstracts* (pp. 102-119). Atlantic Highlands, NJ: Humanities Press.

Kantor, D., & Lehr, W. (1975). *Inside the family.* San Francisco: Jossey-Bass.

Konicek, D. (1976). Marching to a different drummer. In T. Timmerman & J. Ballard (Eds.), *Yearbook in humanistic education.* Amherst, MA: Mandala.

Luce, G. G. (1971). *Body time.* New York: Pantheon Books.

Ornstein, R. E. (1972). *The psychology of consciousness.* San Francisco: W. H. Freeman and Co.

Piaget, J. (1952). *The origins of intelligence in children.* New York: International University Press.

Piaget, J., & Inhelder, B. (1969). *The psychology of the child.* New York: Basic Books.

Schon, D. (1975). Deutero-learning in organizations: Learning for increased effectiveness. *Organizational Dynamics, 4*(1).

Thomas, A., & Chess, S. (1977). *Temperament and development.* New York: Brunner/Mazel.

Von Bertalanffy, L. (1969). General systems theory and psychiatry—An overview. In W. Gray, F. J. Duhl, & N. D. Rizzo (Eds.), *General systems theory and psychiatry.* Boston: Little Brown.

Redefining the Mission
of Family Therapy Training:
Can Our Differentness Make a Difference?

Howard A. Liddle

ABSTRACT. This paper argues for a broadening of the very mission of family therapy training. This challenge to family therapy trainers is organized according to the following four-tiered schema: a) within family therapy, b) between family therapy and psychotherapy, c) among family therapy and other related fields, and d) between family therapy and society. At each of these levels, important questions for family therapy trainers are posed and discussed.

Since the inception of family therapy, the training and supervision subsystem of this field has lagged behind the clinical, theoretical, and research domains. Recently, however, a number of developments in the training area represent significant points of punctuation in the specialty's evolution, perhaps indicating a new era of growth in training and supervision. This trend is evidence by an increasing number of publications[1] in journals, book chapters, and the appearance of comprehensive texts on training family therapists (Duhl, 1983; Flomenhaft & Christ, 1980; Liddle & Saba, in press, a; Liddle, Breunlin & Schwartz, Note 1; Piercy, 1985; Whiffen & Byng-Hall, 1982). There has been, further, a dramatic rise in the volume and quality of presentations on training at the national meetings of family therapy organizations, as well as those of allied disciplines. Professional associations have, in addition, recognized and begun to support organized attention to the training area,[2] a movement that further legitimizes and encourages family therapy training.

When asked about their perceived needs, however, family therapy

The basic content of this chapter comprised an invited address to the Directors of Training Organization of the American Association for Marriage & Family Therapy, October 7, 1983, Washington, D.C. This material also appears in a different form in the text *Training Family Therapists: Creating Contexts of Competence* (N.Y.: Grune & Stratton, in press) by Howard Liddle and George Saba.

Howard A. Liddle, Ed.D., is Director, Behavioral Science Program, Division of Family & Community Medicine, University of California at San Francisco, School of Medicine and San Francisco General Hospital: Director, Family Institute of San Francisco & Faculty, Mental Research Institute, Palo Alto, California.

trainers are not encouraged by recent developments. They express a desire for more practical advances. For example, these trainers specify the need for conceptual frameworks—models of training—as well as increased opportunities for ongoing professional skill development as a supervisor (Saba & Liddle, in press).

Other writings have addressed this necessity of conceptual blueprints that can guide a trainer's actions in the micro (Liddle, 1981, 1982a, 1982b; Liddle & Schwartz, 1983; Liddle & Saba, 1983) and macro (Liddle, 1980; Liddle & Saba, 1982, 1984) moves of training. It is the main premise of this previous work—the principle of isomorphism—that will be touched on and extended in the present chapter. The intent herein is, through using and extending the isomorphism principle, to redraft the framework family therapy trainers have previously used to guide their actions, and more basically, define their mission. The present work argues for a broadening of the very mission of family therapy training. This paper will offer a general framework that considers four distinct but interrelated levels of challenge for family therapy trainers. Within these four levels, specific, difficult questions for trainers will be posed.

A central thrust of my thinking and work in the training area has been the exploration, amplification, and translation of a particular systems phenomenon—isomorphism—into the context of training and supervision. Specifically, I have attempted to outline a conceptual schema for trainers that highlights the points of interconnection of one's therapy and training models, and have outlined ways that this aspect of a system's functioning can be directly translated into action. Using the isomorphism principle as a guide, my colleagues and I have developed a training model that relies heavily on live supervision (Liddle & Schwartz, 1983). Moreover, we have developed a model of training supervisors and therapists interdependently within two training programs (Liddle, Breunlin, Schwartz & Constantine, 1984). In these regards, we have tracked the ways in which the interconnected domains of the therapeutic and training subsystems influence each other, and further, have elaborated the means by which a supervisor uses this knowledge in training. For instance, a supervisor and therapist might conceive of the processes of change in their respective domains in exactly the same way. That is, although the content in each domain might be different, the operational principles of change well may be isomorphic to each other.[3] Thus, consider the supervisor who teaches a structural-strategic approach to therapy that emphasizes the therapist's skillful blending of support and challenge. This model stresses the creation of new workable realities through in-session enactment and between-session directives that attempt to provide a context where alternative ways of experiencing oneself and others can be created. The supervisor may work with this therapist in a parallel way, using these same principles of change in the training context.

The supervisor conceptualizes the tandom application of support and challenge as instrumental to trainee growth. Trainees also perceive a similar process as crucial to their development. In our study of the outcomes of live supervision, trainees overwhelmingly agreed on the need to feel personally supported by their supervisor. At the same time, although they found the stress of the live supervision context and the challenges of the supervisor difficult, they attributed these challenges (e.g., feedback about personal style), as key to their development as therapists (Liddle, Davidson & Barrett, Note 2).

Our ability to understand and map out the isomorphic processes between training and therapy is greatly enhanced by our interactional framework. Referred to in different quarters as the systemic or contextual paradigm, the ecosystemic or cybernetic epistemology, or the interpersonal or interactional view, this frame of reference prevents family therapy from being narrowly categorized simply as a technique. Instead family therapy is seen as an orientation to human problems.

From this vantage point, a therapist does not only help couples and families solve problems, come to grips with their past, or behave in new ways. In addition, clinical work has an epistemology-shaping component. Whether our therapy directly teaches families a new epistemology of life or interpersonal relations (i.e., an alternate acceptable way of making sense of the world), or arranges in-the-room and between-session contexts in which families discover and create new epistemologies, it is important that family members develop this alternate vision and set of beliefs, along with corresponding behavior change. Isomorphically, then, the essence of training can be considered the same. That is, training challenges and alters trainee's previous conceptions of human behavior, while developing skills that translate this broadened perspective into clinically useful alternatives. If therapy's goal can be generically thought of as the contextualization of our clients, the goal of training likewise can be considered the contextualization of our trainees.

Such an isomorphic perspective on therapy and supervision logically leads to a set of problem areas that should be of the highest priority to family therapy trainers. These concerns are summed up in the following four questions:

First, at the level of the family therapy field itself, we must begin to question the degree and forms of dialogue and interchange available. More basically, we might question many of our field's key players' capacity to engage in dialogue, especially in situations where saving face or maintaining one's status appears to be primary. As many have observed, the stuggle to create and differentiate the various schools of thought—''the movement to stake a territory'' (Sluzki, 1983)—can have isolating, stultifying effects. Thus, within family therapy, how do we interpret and decide to accept or challenge, what many have felt to be the artificial or overly rigid boundaries demarcating present points of view?

Second, at the level of the family therapy field in relation to the profession of psychotherapy and field of mental health, we can ask: to what extent have we influenced our colleagues in psychotherapy, and what impact has the family therapy viewpoint had in the course of psychotherapy's development? Conversely, to what extent have we allowed ourselves to be influenced by other developing ideas from the broadly-based psychotherapy field? In effect, we must examine the boundary around family therapy.

Third, at the level of family therapy in relation to other fields that, in their own ways, deal with systems ideas: to what extent have we influenced domains outside of therapy, and in turn comprehended and utilized these domains to enhance and refine our own interpretation of systems thinking? Here, of course, we are examining the boundary between family therapy/psychotherapy and related systems fields.

The *fourth* level concerns the content to which systems thinking has been incorporated into our society at large. Have we influenced the ways in which our popular culture views human relationships and problems? And, more basically, do we have a responsibility for such a grand, or what some might call grandiose, endeavor? If there can be a "Greening of America" (Reich, 1970), can there be a "contextualizing" of the same (or even broader) territory?

THE FOUR LEVELS OF FOCUS

Within Family Therapy. The schools of thought within the field have been involved in an internally focused, self-defining, generative, and in Koestler's (1978) terms, self-assertive undertaking.[4] The proponents of these singular viewpoints have been devoted to *intra-model* specification, elaboration, and experimentation. While understandable in the developmental scheme of things, this self-assertive style would do well to move more toward dialogue and integration. New forums of interchange designed in the field, while far from completely satisfying, are moving in a more enlightened direction. Innovative programming alone, however, will not guarantee the success of an interactive conference. Many presenters are not accustomed to or adept at dialoguing with their colleagues. Even conferences with an excellent structure (e.g., different therapists interviewing the same case), can fail when clinicians do not discuss directly with each other the same stimuli. Similarly, problems arise when there is no conference chair or moderator to encourage and organize such interaction.

Increasingly, we hear the call for an integration of points of view in our field. Although we can enumerate inherent conceptual dangers and practical problems in any integrative effort (Liddle, 1982c), not the least of which is the degree to which therapists underestimate its difficulty, the spirit of integration is here to stay, and should be considered well-intentioned and worthwhile (Lebow, 1984). Trainers will be faced consistently with the problems of integrating family therapy models, since trainees are interested in integrative approaches, as well as the "pure," "single-theory" models.

My own work along these lines has involved generating guidelines for judging successful and unsuccessful application of an integrative structural-strategic theory (Liddle, 1985), as well as the construction of a theoretical scaffolding with generic constructs for this approach (Liddle, 1984b). These efforts are posed in the spirit of previous recommendations for trainers' (and therapists') articulation of their own essential presuppositions about the training enterprise in general and change in particular. This work is basic to the clarification and construction of personal, evolving models of therapy and training (Liddle, 1985). This activity is, simultaneously, indispensable to individual practice, as well as recursive and regenerative. In sum, the *Within Family Therapy* question relates to the issue of boundaries "inside" the field. These sometimes overly constricting boundaries separate the schools of thought and their proponents from meaningful, potentially enriching and synergistic interchange.

Further, boundary difficulties often exist among the domains of research, clinical practice, and theory development. It is often difficult to remember that trainers in particular are always functioning, though not formally nor with official labels, at the intersections of these interlinked areas. Trainers are researchers in the sense of monitoring the outcome of their training with trainees and with the cases their trainees see. Trainers are concerned with clinical practice since they are never far from the clinical material of their trainees. And trainers are theoreticians in the sense that they teach particular theoretical models, as well as the integration of these models, to their trainees. Consequently, trainers need to master not only the various approaches and their points of interconnection and overlap, but also need to define the guidelines for building an integrative model[6]—a task just beginning in the family therapy field.[7]

Family Therapy as a Subsystem Within Psychotherapy. This area of inquiry challenges family therapists' isolationist stance vis-à-vis other spheres of psychotherapy. Historically, family therapists have been the mavericks of the therapy world, and in recent times, perhaps have taken up where the behaviorists left off. Thus far at least, family therapists have opted, in a way that is understandable and justifiable in developmental terms,[8] for self-assertion at the expense of integration. Apparently, we have been more suited to the role of outsiders—the critical, anti-establishment, vocal minority, adept at defining what we are by declaring what we are not.

In relation, particularly, to the recent epistemological renewal in our field, we might pose the following question. If we professionally *and* personally believe in the systems viewpoint and what it represents—nonlinearity, interdependence, interconnectedness—than can we continue our separatist policy in relation to the mental health world? To remain unconnected, or as Bowen might say, cut off, from the rest of psychotherapy because "our ideas are in need of further development" gives an overly pessimistic assessment of family therapy's development, and additionally, ignores the potential gains from such synergy-producing encounters.

It will take maturity to consider the complaints leveled against family therapy from other quarters. Arrogance, aloofness, manipulativeness, conceptual and technical rigidity—these are, as we know, partial, relativistic descriptions of one side of reality. Nonetheless, they represent what others define as real—as their versions of and reactions to the family therapy movement. To dismiss these perceptions as unfounded and irrelevant, especially at this stage of our field's development, misses the point of what it means to be a family therapist. Thus far, we have been able to be unconcerned about our profile in the broad community of therapists. This posture has an anachronistic and strangely contradictory ring to it—to ignore our position in this broader context is to behave in an acontextual manner—the very way of being we seek to change with our trainees and clinical families.

Similarly, we must begin to question seriously our degree of influence in the mental health community. It is easy to dismiss this concern with a plea to consider how far family therapy has come, and certainly we must view our current degree of influence[9] in perspective. The family therapy viewpoint is undoubtedly more visible and accepted today than in the past, even a decade ago. But to get a distinctly different reading of family therapy's posture than is obtainable at our own meetings (e.g., American Association for Marriage and Family Therapy, American Family Therapy Association), one can simply attend, or better still, present on family therapy at conferences of the American Psychological Association, American Psychiatric Association, or National Association of Social Workers. We may be adept at talking with our family therapy colleagues, but considerably less able to move as easily in the circles of our original disciplines. There exists within these primarily non-family therapy contexts a tremendous potential for influence, refinement and enrichment. Unfortunately, family therapists in these settings often exhibit an attitude of superiority that when in full bloom, manifested itself in the troublesome systemic chic (Liddle & Saba, 1981, 1981b) and epistobabble (Coyne, 1982; Coyne, Denner & Ransom, 1983) phenomena some of us find so objectionable.

One major resource or means of intervention at this interface of family therapy and mental health is the product of our training efforts—our family therapy trainees. Previous work (Liddle, 1978) detailed some of the consequences of trainees' adopting a systemic perspective in a university psychology department. This previous paper also attempted, from the trainers' perspective, to address the problems of effectively teaching this minority view in an unsympathetic setting. The notion of *preparing* trainees for the consequences of their change to the family therapy view, thus became a major focus of this work.

One might legitimately ask, is not good training and supervision in and of itself enough, and will not these systems ideas we teach trainees generalize to the trainees'/therapists' work domains as well? In most cases, the answer is a resounding no. Our continuing study of live supervision outcomes reveals that trainees want and need help in putting their training into practice (Liddle et al., Note 2).

Trainees' work contexts are not the only problems in the relationship of family therapy to the mental health establishment. A therapist in a training program is particularly vulnerable to unrealistic expectations regarding how his/her colleagues "should" respond to family therapy. Training programs are distinct cultures, with attendant values and an intensity of their own. Trainees often are insensitive to the ways in which their excitement about learning something new is not shared by non-family therapy colleagues. A conscious "toning down" of overly zealous conversation tactics, then, may be a realistic and worthy goal of training, especially in the early stages.

The general issue of family therapy's link with psychotherapy can be complicated further by a short-term and narrowly-construed vision of training. Although it is true that in some ways we all will always remain learners of our complex craft, trainees do not remain trainees forever. Our trainees become one of us, full-fledged members of a chosen profession. Of course, a professional hierarchy often develops around such variables as experience, work setting, visibility and reputation, publications, degree, etc. Yet there is an undeniable commonality among all those clinicians who call themselves systems thinkers or family therapists. In an international survey of over 1000 American Association for Marriage and Family Therapy (AAMFT)—approved supervisors and American Family Therapy Association (AFTA) members, the respondents resoundingly echoed a uniform assessment of their primary function and difficulty as teachers of family therapy: the facilitation of the systemic view with their trainees. This research suggests that supervisors realize full well that they are not merely producing a new breed of technologists (Saba & Liddle, in press). These teachers of family therapy are aware that they are intervening at an epistemological level with their trainees—not only about therapeutic matters, but about the very way in which these trainees/therapists construe everyday life and human relationships.

Is it not also our assumption, perhaps not always in the foreground, that these trainees/therapists will, in their own way and time, carry forth to others this systemic view? If this is so, it would seem that the field and our trainees would be well served by training that is sensitive to how best to communicate an interactional view. Such training should prepare trainees for the personal and contextual consequences of change to the systemic view. This training also should address the ways in which family therapists serve as intentional and unintentional systemic ambassadors, as well as provide a means by which this role can be effectively implemented.

My position argues for an expansion of the trainer's conception of *professional preparation*. It includes attention to the political side of a family therapist's professional socialization. It is insufficient only to assist trainees in personally defining and generating a plan for continuing professional development (i.e., self-supervision, self-renewal as a therapist, development of a personal, evolving model of therapy), although these must be considered important training goals. Historically, and in a contemporary sense, the politics of family therapy have been an essential aspect of articulating and practicing the systemic view (Haley, 1976). The premise herein is not that adequate preparation can prevent difficulties for trainees in these areas. It is rather than such difficulties are natural and inevitable, and the concept of political sensitization, instead of preventing problems, prepares trainees to deal with these inevitabilities in a more informed manner. Trainees should be taught, directly and indirectly, that sensitivity to the politics of family therapy is an important aspect of a systemic view.

Family Therapy and Other Systems Fields

At the third level, we can consider how family therapy conceptually and practically interconnects with other systems-oriented fields. Certainly our tradition has been an interdisciplinary one. Systems-oriented professionals within and outside the mental health community have found common interests, orientations, and thinking under the family therapy rubric. The theoretical foundations of our field have relied extensively on principles and concepts from such diverse fields of study as biology, cybernetics, information and communication theory, among other. A recent movement in family therapy, sometimes referred to as the epistemologic renewal, has challenged us to reexamine our presuppositional beliefs about fundamental human and clinical issues. In this sense, the resurgence of interest in epistemology, and theory in general, has been productive and proactive. It has encouraged us to focus on the processes and difficulties of defining the systemic paradigm in family therapy (Liddle, 1984; in press).

This trend has not been without its critics (Coyne, 1982; Coyne, Denner & Ransom, 1983; Liddle & Saba, 1981a, 1981b). These critics of the epistemologic renewal have helped us question the manner in which we apply and sometimes misapply metaphors, concepts, and principles from other fields. We often have overused and misused the principle of interconnection between fields in the quest to become more sophisticated. To overemploy or misapply constructs from other fields is to violate one of the most essential premises of our work—the notion of contextual relativity. To translate these analogies is to chop their ecology, as the saying goes in our field—to be insensitive to their idiosyncratic meaning in their context-of-origin. Perhaps Kuhn's (1970) suggestion of the benefits of a cross-context and paradigm translation and interpretation process has relevance here.

Despite the ease with which ideas for such conceptual cross-fertilization can be made, there remains the issues of what specific kinds of contexts can be constructed to fit these goals, and further, what are some of the problems that will arise when these forums are held? A recent conference sponsored by the Mental Research Institute, "Maps of the World" illustrates our developmental stage in the process of interchange with related fields. This conference brought together family therapists with cyberneticians and others involved in the development of systems theory with nonhuman systems. A major part of the program involved dialogue among the panel (clinicians and nonclinician-systems experts), and between the panel and audience. Those therapists with an expectation of a high level of integration and synthesis of systems theory in the clinical and nonclinical realm (i.e., belief that there were immediately translatable, or *worse,* already translated answers from nonclinical fields) left the most disappointed. Therapists with less utopian expectations about the amount or degree of *immediately clinically usable* material that would evolve from these dialogues seemed more satisfied with the conference's avant garde focus.

Since family therapy trainers work at the intersection of theory, practice, and research, we have a role in supporting these kinds of events. We also should help therapists and trainees remember that explorations such as these, although needed, will not always bear immediate pragmatic results.

These experimental contexts raise the question of how the systems view is learned. We know that our knowledge of systems comes from many sources, including our own families. Many therapists, through life experiences and intellectual pursuits, discover the systemic paradigm long before hearing the term "family therapy."

As trainers we are on the lookout for ways to facilitate this vision with our trainees (Henry & Storm, 1984). One useful training tool, for example, is Capra's (1975) *Tao of Physics.* Capra sketches the epistemologic parallels between the eastern religions and the new physics, emphasizing the systemic nature of each. In a text of this nature, although never mentioning family therapy, therapists can gain a deeper, richer comprehension of the contextual view. Capra's (1982) other major book, *The Turning Point,* can have similar integrative effects with trainees (Liddle, 1982d). Capra examines the prevailing world views in such fields as medicine, economics, politics and government, and psychology and traces the ways that systems thinking has or has not been introduced.

Personal involvement in other spheres of systems activity also can provide profound learning experiences, both for us and others. Many family therapists currently work, for example, in fields such as family medicine, where their challenging roles as teacher, supervisor (Liddle & Saba, Reference note) and consultant (Bloch, 1984) allow them to articulate the systems viewpoint to the medical world. The possibilities, benefits, and difficulties of family therapists assuming such positions in a variety of fields are just now receiving the exploration they merit.[10] This expansion of the roles of the family therapist is a rich area of inquiry, especially for family therapy trainers.

Beyond Family Therapy: The Systems Perspective In Society. How do we define the limits or boundaries of our role as family therapists? Do we have any obligation to society to forward the systems philosophy? Pragmatically, therapists might engage in this broadly-based pursuit in order to advance the legitimization of family therapy. From an ethical or moral perspective, the systems framework might be seen as a paradigm offering alternative perceptual and problem solving possibilities to a struggling world (Bohm, 1980; Bursztajan et al., 1982; Capra, 1975, 1982; Dossey, 1982; Jantsch, 1980; Jantsch & Waddington, 1976; Pelletier, 1979; Prigogine & Stengers, 1984; Toffler, 1983).

One's position on this matter is, in part, based on assumptions about the potential applicability of the systems view. If its usefulness is assessed to be fairly circumscribed, its translation into other domains would seem inappropriate. Conversely, if the paradigm's principles seem transferable and capable of being modified to a variety of contexts, its migration in a macrosystemic, transcontextual direction would be more likely accepted.[11]

Another factor affecting our thinking about the potential role of systems thinking in society is the way we define our role as a professional. From one perspective, we have taken the designation "family therapy" too literally. In a sense, we seem to have moved the locus of pathology from the unit of the individual to the family. To what degree do we now blame the family in a perhaps more sophisticated, but isomorphically similar way to the way that individuals traditionally were deemed as dysfunctional? Further, do we only define our role as therapists in terms of working "on" these dysfunctional family units? If we define problems in interactional, mutually causative, interdependent ways, is not our unit of assessment and intervention expandable to larger and larger systems? To speculate in this direction, however, is to inevitably experience the valid doubts about the feasibility, complexity, and difficulty of this vision-expanding task. As the saying goes: After all, what can one person do? (And besides, where would one begin?)

Related to the deliteralization of family therapy ideas are our beliefs and values about such matters as prevention and popularization. Generally, prevention has not achieved widespread attention or adoption by most therapists. Although psychoeducational therapies are achieving some recognition in family therapy, the "therapeutic" and educational models of change have been conceived as separate entities, hierarchically organized in terms of their perceived attractiveness. Therapists want to do therapy, not provide educational guidance. Of course, the fact that much of therapy has educative, information-providing components does not seem to matter. Therapists interested in preventative work with non-clinical families, for instance, are often relegated to second rate status. The family and couple enrichment movement has suffered by comparison to the family therapy field, which was profiled and defined from the beginning as exciting.

Introducing systems ideas into our society can have preventative as well as problem-solving possibilities. In the field of international relations, for example, a systems view facilitates a more-of-the-same analysis of nationalistic rhetoric and arms buildup (Moley, in press). To see such buildup as symmetrical escalation is a first step in possibly breaking this dangerous cycle.

The matter of translating scientific or technical findings and concepts into the public domain has been a controversial one across fields of study. The majority of professionals within any given discipline seem to disregard, downplay, or downright denigrate the popularization of their field's research or clinical findings. Charges of oversimplification, misrepresentation, financial gain, and/or personal promotion are levied against many of those who have chosen to write and talk about their/our craft to the public.

Our suspicion and lack of respect for many of these popularizers, however, is sometimes warranted. We all have different tolerance levels for such activities. For some, the breaking point comes with Dr. Joyce Brothers' appearance on the Gong Show, or Virginia Satir's Caribbean Cruises. For others, the point of no return might be a Leo Buscaglia hugfest or the hottest new self-proclaimed self-help expert on the talk show stump. But what about less easy targets? What about those professionals with a sincere belief in the need for popularization and information transmission efforts *and* solid content in a respectable package to back it up?

Obviously, there are no easy answers. A concern of mine involves prominent news persons interviewing guest experts in an attempt to uncover *the single cause* of crime, delinquency, alcoholism, drug abuse, inflation, unemployment, international strife, arms proliferation and the like. Is the prevailing epistemology's assumption that the "common man" is not capable of understanding or dealing with the complexity and ambiguity associated with, for example, nonlineal, mutually-influencing conceptions of causality?

A typical issue of the Sunday *New York Times* magazine recently featured two interesting articles: one on architectural trends, the other on borderline personalities. The architectural piece was written from a systems perspective—a vantage point that understood and communicated the idea of context. Sad but true, the borderline piece, like most mental health articles in popular publications, reflected an acontextual way of understanding humans and their problems. The architecture article, on the other hand, magnificently dealt with the notion of a building's *relationship* to its natural or neighborhood ecology. In this example, the spokesperson for systemic thinking was not a mental health expert but an architecture critic. The continued low profile of literate systems oriented mental health professionals in the public domain is a problem the family theapy field has not been willing to address.

SUMMARY AND CONCLUSIONS

Family therapy is at a critical juncture in its evolution. Many schools of thought exist; their methods and concepts increasingly are being specified. Research is well underway, and although early in its development, is beginning to validate the effectiveness of systems-oriented approaches. A training technology exists and general frameworks or models of training have progressed beyond their crudest beginnings. Still, with all these hallmarks of progress, the family therapy field's influence in mental health and society at large must now be called into question. This paper has organized a challenge to family therapy trainers according to a four-tiered schema: within family therapy, family therapy and psychotherapy, family therapy and other systems related fields, and family therapy and society. The major implications of this challenge can be reformulated and put forth in the following:

1. We have had a propensity to talk *past* or *down to,* rather than *with* each other. The field's capacity to converse with itself, to truly engage in a dialogue about matter of both content and politics (i.e., about the "big questions" of influence, the meaning of the systemic view, etc.) seems basic if the field is ever to influence others.
2. The present challenge aims to ask: what are the big questions for

trainers, and for the field? I have postulated, here and elsewhere, that these matters can be grouped into categories such as:

    a. Integration of theories/schools of thought (i.e., rules relating to theory-building and the construction of personal, evolving models of therapy and training);

    b. continuing professional development (i.e., innovative programming in conferences and the creation of new forums in which genuine professional growth can occur);

    c. interpentration of practice, theory, and research (i.e., developing the specific ways in which these domains interconnect and relate in one's work);

    d. redefinition of training and the role of a trainer (i.e., expanding the previous narrow definition of clinical preparation).

3. The final challenge falls into the Beyond Family Therapy (Liddle, 1984a) category. It asserts that a broadening, deliteralization, and redefinition should occur. It is the old "Whither Family Therapy?" question posed from a new developmental stage. Today, the answers to this timeless question, as well as the generation of new questions are needed. We have just begun to explore the full implications of the systemic view. Some of our questions will take us far from where we think we began as family therapists. Perhaps, though, the answers we find will feel like home.

> We shall not cease from exploration
> And the end of all our exploring
> Will be to arrive where we started
> And know the place for the first time
>
> *T. S. Eliot*

FOOTNOTES

1. There are now in excess of 225 publications, scattered in a wide variety of collected readings and journals, specifically addressing some aspect of family therapy training.

2. The American Association for Marriage & Family Therapy (AAMFT) has organized two independently functioning bodies, the Commission on Accreditation and the Commission on Supervision to address different aspects of training. The AAMFT has also appointed a Task Force on the Recognition, Regulation, and Legitimization of Marital and Family Therapy. Additionally, the American Family Therapy Association has authorized the formation of a Task Force on Family Therapy Training.

3. isomorph: *iso:* similar or same
              morph: structure

4. Koestler's holon concept (holos: "whole;" prot*on*/neutr*on:* "part") has enjoyed considerable pragmatic and conceptual utility. With this term, Koestler sought to provide the perceptual flexibility needed in systems analysis. Humans and other systems, from Koestler's vantage point,

can be seen as holons—organisms having two opposite, but complementary, tendencies or potentials: an *integrative* tendency to function as part of the larger whole, and a *self-assertive* tendency to preserve its *individual autonomy.* Koestler's concept, in his own words, "is meant to supply the missing link between atomism and holism, and to supplant the dualistic way of thinking in terms of 'parts' and 'wholes,' which is so deeply engrained in our mental habits by a multi-level, stratified approach (Koestler, 1978, p. 293). For Koestler, parts and wholes, in the absolute senses in which they are usually referred, do not exist in life. The model of integrative and self-assertive tendencies of systems has been quite useful in the formulation of the questions posed and the dimensions outlined in this paper.

5. The Philadelphia Child Guidance Clinic's Dialogues and Trialogues conferences of 1981 and 1982; the Mental Research Institute's Biennial Conference of 1983 ("Maps of the Mind: Maps of the World"); and the Houston-Galveston Family Institute's Conference on Epistemology in 1983 are but a few of these interaction prompting attempts of note.

6. This is not meant to imply that our quest should be to build one integrative, supermodel—an approach that encompasses all other models. A series of integrative models is a more reasonable and likely pursuit. In Jantsch's (1980) terms, there is a need in a number of fields of inquiry for an *ecology* or *pluralism of models*—a cluster of interlinked yet distinct (in our case integrative) frameworks, each having its own domain of applicability and effectiveness.

7. Much recent work in the field (e.g., Gurman, 1981; Liddle, 1984, 1985; Stanton, 1984) has dealt with issues such as the need for consistency in integrative models, specific guidelines for making clinical decisions within a model, contextual and personal variations involved in constructing integrative models, and the possibilities offered by the utilization of metatheoretical constructs that can link different theoretical approaches in a unified whole.

8. Developmental reframing, whether it be in relation to a patient, family, or entire field, seems to be a useful attribution for why something appears to be, at present, problematic. Here the tone is intended to be that the self-assertive mode has been appropriate at previous development stages, but should it continue without increased integrative tendencies, the field's growth would be retarded.

9. Influence is meant in the broadest possible sense; it should not be construed as an unidirectional process with the goal of converting those unfortunates who do not share our view of the world and therapy. Its use here implies a reciprocal kind of influence in which differing points of view, through their interaction, will each help to clarify and shape the other position.

10. For example, a forthcoming text, *The family therapist as consultant: New applications of systems theory,* edited by Lyman Wynne and associates at Rochester (Guilford Press), will offer a broadly based look at how the skills and perspectives of family therapists are used in a multitude of contexts, including courts, police, schools, and medicine, among others.

11. A recently published book by J. Schwartzman (1984) and a theme issue of the *Journal of Strategic & Systemic Therapies* (Saba, in press) were devoted to the isomorphic application of systems ideas acrosss a variety of settings and content domains.

REFERENCES

Bloch, D. (1984). The family therapist as health care consultant. *Family Systems Medicine, 2,* 161-169.

Bohm, D. (1980). *Wholeness and the implicate order.* London: Routledge & Kegan Paul.

Bursztajan, H., Feinbloom, R., Hamm, R., & Brodsky, A. (1981). *Medical choices, medical chances.* New York: Delta.

Capra, F. (1982). *The turning point.* New York: Simon & Schuster.

Capra, F. (1975). *The tao of physics.* Boulder, CO: Shambhala.

Coyne, J. (1982). A brief introduction to epistobabble. *The Family Therapy Networker, 6*(4), 27-28.

Coyne, J., Denner, B., & Ransom, D. (1982). Undressing the fashionable mind. *Family Process, 21,* 391-396.

Dossey, L. (1982). *Space, time & medicine.* Boulder, CO: Shanbhala.

Duhl, B. (1983). *From the inside out.* New York: Brunner/Mazel.

Flomenhaft, K., & Christ, A. (1980). *The challenge of family therapy.* New York: Plenum.

Gurman, A. (1981). Integrative marital therapy; Toward the development of an interpersonal approach. In S. Budman (Ed.), *Forms of brief therapy*. New York: Guilford.

Haley, J. (1976). *Problem solving therapy*. San Francisco: Jossey-Bass.

Henry, P., & Storm, C. (1984). The training metamorphosis: Teaching systemic thinking in family therapy programs. *Journal of Strategic and Systemic Therapies, 3*, 41-49.

Jantsch, E. (1980). *The self-organizing universe*. Elmsford, NY: Pergamon.

Jantsch, E., & Waddington, C. (Eds.). (1975). *Evolution and consciousness: Human systems in transition*. Reading, MA: Addison-Wesley.

Koestler, A. (1978). *Janus: A summing up*. New York: Random House.

Kuhn, T. S. (1970). *The structure of scientific revolutions*. Chicago: University of Chicago Press (Second Edition).

Lebow, J. (1984). On the value of integrating approaches to family therapy. *Journal of Marital and Family Therapy, 10*, 127-138.

Liddle, H. A. (1978). The emotional and political hazards of teaching and learning family therapy. *Family Therapy, 5*, 1-12.

Liddle, H. A. (1980). On teaching a contextual or systemic therapy: Training content, goals and methods. *American Journal of Family Therapy, 8*, 58-69.

Liddle, H. A. (1981). Keeping abreast of developments in the family therapy field: The use of "concept cards" in clinical practice. In A. Gurman (Ed.), *Questions and answers in family therapy* (Vol. 1). New York: Brunner/Mazel.

Liddle, H. A. (1982a). Family therapy training: Current issues, future trends. *International Journal of Family Therapy, 4*, 81-97(c).

Liddle, H. A. (1982b). In the mind's eye: Use of visual and auditory imagery in creating therapeutic and supervisory realities. In A. Gurman (Ed.), *Questions and answers in family therapy* (Vol. 2). New York: Brunner/Mazel.

Liddle, H. A. (1982c). On the problems of eclecticism: A call for epistemologic clarification and human-scale theories. *Family Process, 21*, 243-250.

Liddle, H. A. (1982d). Review of Capra, F. *The turning point*. In *Journal of Marital and Family Therapy, 8*, 474-475.

Liddle, H. A., Bruenlin, D., & Schwartz, R. (In preparation). *Handbook of family therapy training*. New York: Guilford Press.

Liddle, H. A., Davidson, G. S., & Barrett, M. J. (In preparation). Outcomes of live supervision: Trainee perspectives. In H. A. Liddle et al: (Eds.), *Handbook of family therapy training and supervision*. New York: Guilford Press.

Liddle, H. A., & Saba, G. (Manuscript submitted for publication). Broadening the focus of behavioral science in family practice.

Liddle, H. A. (1984a). Beyond family therapy I: Design for evolution, *Family Therapy News*, January, 1984; Beyond family therapy II: Personal definitions, *Family Therapy News*, March, 1984; Beyond family therapy III: Definition difficulties, *Family Therapy News*, May, 1984; Beyond family therapy IV: Implementation difficulties, *Family Therapy News*, July, 1984; Beyond family therapy V: A political analogy, *Family Therapy News*, September, 1984(a).

Liddle, H. A. (1984b). Toward a dialectical-contextual-coevolutionary translation of structural-strategic therapy. *Journal of Strategic and Systemic Therapies, 4*(3), 64-78(b).

Liddle, H. A. (1985). Five factors of failure in Structural-Strategic family therapy: A contextual construction. In S. Coleman (Ed.), *Failures in family therapy*. New York: Guilford Press.

Liddle, H. A. (In press). Reflections of a family therapy trainer. In D. Efron (Ed.), *Strategic and systemic therapies*. New York: Brunner/Mazel.

Liddle, H. A., & Saba, G. (1981a). Systemic Chic: Family therapy's new wave. *Journal of Strategic and Systemic Therapies, 1*(2), 36-39(a).

Liddle, H. A., & Saba, G. (1981b). Systemic chic II: Can family therapy maintain its floy floy? *Journal of Strategic and Systemic Therapies, 1*(2), 40-43(b).

Liddle, H. A., & Saba, G. (1982). On teaching family therapy at the introductory level: A conceptual model emphasizing a pattern which connects training and therapy. *Journal of Marital and Family Therapy, 8*, 63-72.

Liddle, H. A., & Saba, G. W. (1983). On context replication: The isomorphic nature of training and therapy. *Journal of Strategic and Systemic Therapies, 2*(3), 3-11.

Liddle, H. A., & Saba, G. W. (1984). The isomorphic nature of training and therapy: Epistemologic foundation for a Structural-Strategic training paradigm. In J. Schwartzman (Ed.), *Families and other systems*. New York: Guilford Press.

Liddle, H. A., & Saba, G. (In press, a). *Training family therapists: Creating contexts of competence.* New York: Grune and Stratton.

Liddle, H. A., Breunlin, D., Schwartz, R., & Constantine, J. (1984). Training family therapy supervisors: Issues of content, form and context. *Journal of Marital and Family Therapy, 10,* 139-150.

Liddle, H. A. & Schwartz, R. (1983). Live supervision/consultation: Pragmatic and conceptual guidelines for family therapy trainers, *Family Process, 22,* 477-490.

Moley, V. (In press). An interactional perspective of international disorders. *Journal of Strategic and Systemic Therapies.*

Pelletier, K. (1979). *Holistic medicine.* New York: Dell.

Piercy, F. (1985). *Family therapy education and supervision.* New York: Haworth.

Prigogine, I., & Stengers, I. (1984). *Order out of chaos: Man's new dialogue with nature.* New York: Bantam.

Reich, C. (1970). *The greening of America.* New York: Random House.

Saba, G. (In press). Theme issue on the application of systems ideas across content areas and contexts. *Journal of Strategic & Systemic Therapies.*

Saba, G. W., & Liddle, H. A. (In press). Perceptions of professional needs, practice patterns and critical issues facing family therapy trainers and supervisors. *American Journal of Family Therapy.*

Schwartzman, J. (Ed.), (1984). *Families and other systems.* New York: Guilford.

Sluzki, C. (1983). How to stake a territory in the field of family therapy in three easy lessons. *Journal of Marital and Family Therapy, 9,* 235-238.

Stanton, M. D. (1984). Fusion, compression, diversion, and the workings of paradox: A theory of therapeutic/systemic change. *Family Process, 23,* 135-168.

Toffler, A. (1983). *Previews and premises.* New York: William Morrow.

Whiffen, M., & Byng-Hall, J. (1982). *Family therapy supervision.* London: Academic.

RESOURCE SECTIONS

Commission on Accreditation for Marriage and Family Therapy Education

ACCREDITED GRADUATE PROGRAMS

ABILENE CHRISTIAN UNIVERSITY
Marriage and Family Institute
Abilene, TX 79699

Paul B. Faulkner, Ph.D.
(915) 677-1911

BRIGHAM YOUNG UNIVERSITY
Marriage and Family Therapy Program
Provo, UT 84602

Robert F. Stahmann, Ph.D.
(801) 374-1211

EAST TEXAS STATE UNIVERSITY
Dept. of Counseling and Guidance
Commerce, TX 75428

Pat Lutz, Ed.D.
(214) 886-5631, 5637

GEORGIA STATE UNIVERSITY
Family Psychology
Atlanta, GA 30303

Luciano L'Abate
(404) 658-2283

KANSAS STATE UNIVERSITY
Dept. of Family and Child Development
Just Hall
Manhattan, KS 66506

Candyce S. Russell, Ph.D.
(913) 532-5510

LOMA LINDA UNIVERSITY
Dept. of Marriage and Family Therapy
Loma Linda, CA 92354

Antonius Brandon, Ph.D.
(714) 824-4547
      814-0800 ex. 4547

NORTHERN ILLINOIS UNIVERSITY
Dept. of Home Economics
DeKalb, IL 60155

Connie Salts, Ph.D.
(815) 753-1196

PURDUE UNIVERSITY
Marriage and Family Therapy Center
CDFS Bldg.
West Lafayette, IN 47907

Douglas Sprenkle, Ph.D.
(317) 494-2939

SOUTHERN CONNECTICUT STATE
Counseling and School Psychology Dept.
501 Cresent Street
New Haven, CT 06515

Rocco Orlando, Ph.D.
(203) 397-4574, 4580

TEXAS TECH UNIVERSITY
Dept. of Home and Family Life
P.O. Box 4170
Lubbock, TX 79409

Harvey Joanning, Ph.D.
(806) 742-3000

UNIVERSITY OF BRIDGEPORT
College of Health Sciences
Bridgeport, CT 06601

Gerald Arndt, Ed.D.
(203) 576-4173

UNIVERSITY OF HOUSTON
  AT CLEAR LAKE
Behavioral Sciences Program
2700 Bay Area Blvd.
Houston, TX 77058

Linda Bell, Ph.D.
(713) 488-9236

UNIVERSITY OF CONNECTICUT
School of Family Studies
U-58
Storrs, CT 06268

Robert Ryder, Ph.D.
(203) 486-4633

UNIVERSITY OF MARYLAND
Dept. of Family and Community Dev.
College Park, MD 20742

Ned L. Gaylin, Ph.D.
(301) 454-2142

UNIVERSITY OF SOUTHERN
  CALIFORNIA
Dept. of Sociology
J.P. Human Relations Center
725 West 27th Street
Los Angeles, CA 90007

Carlfred Broderick, Ph.D.
(213) 743-2137

UNIVERSITY OF
  WISCONSIN-STOUT
School of Education and Human
Services
Menamonie, WI 54751

Charles Barnard, Ed.D.
(715) 232-2404

VIRGINIA TECH UNIVERSITY
Marriage and Family Therapy Program
Dept. of Family and Child Development
Blacksburg, VA 24061

James F. Keller, Ph.D.
(703) 961-7201

ACCREDITED POST DEGREE PROGRAMS

ACKERMAN INSTITUTE OF
  FAMILY THERAPY
148 East 78th Street
New York, NY 10021

Robert Simon, M.D.
(212) 879-4900

CALIFORNIA FAMILY
STUDY CENTER
4400 Riverside Drive
Burbank, CA 91505

Edwin S. Cox, Ph.D.
(213) 843-0711

CLSC-METRO (PEEL CENTRE)
Marriage Counseling Service
1550 de Mainsonneuve St. West
Suite 400
Montreal, Quebec, H3G IN2

Sharon Bond, M.S.W.
935-2179

FAMILY AND CHILDREN
SERVICES OF GREATER ST.
LOUIS
2650 Olive Street
St. Louis, MO 63103

Paul Reed, M.S.W.
(314) 371-6500

FAMILY INSTITUTE OF
WESTCHESTER
147 Archer Ave.
Mt. Vernon, NY 10550

Elizabeth Carter
(914) 699-4300

MARRIAGE COUNCIL OF
PHILADELPHIA
4025 Chestnut Street
Philadelphia, PA 19104

Ellen Berman, M.D.
(215) 382-6680

FAMILY SERVICE OF MILWAUKEE
Box 08434
Milwaukee, WI 53208

Judith E. Tietyen, A.C.S.W.
(414) 342-4560

Book Reviews on Family Therapy Training and Supervision

FAMILY THERAPY SUPERVISION: RECENT DEVELOPMENTS IN PRACTICE. Whiffen, R., & Byng-Hall, J. (Eds.). (1982). *New York: Grune & Stratton. 217 pp., $29.50.*

Future historians of family therapy will acclaim this book for two distinctions. First, it is the first book to specifically address the topic of family therapy supervision. Second, the editors have captured the theory and practice of supervision in the late seventies and early eighties in one cross-sectional slice. The value of this volume for the contemporary reader is the breadth of family therapy supervision theory and technique presented.

In 1979, the Tavistock Clinic in London hosted the International Forum for Family Therapy Trainers. From an array of divergent contexts, the participants expressed an interest in new ways of conducting supervision and in sharing their ideas with a wider audience. The result is an internationally-flavored collection of 19 papers on family therapy supervision. The editors instructed contributors to: (a) describe their supervision style, (b) describe its relationship to a therapeutic approach, and (c) provide examples of family therapy supervision practice. Training centers in Italy, West Germany, the United Kingdom, Canada, and the United States provided such accounts of their work. Rosemary Whiffen and John Byng-Hall have somewhat loosely organized these informative articles into the following five sections: evolution of supervision, special techniques, the learning process, supervisory methods related to specific conceptual frameworks, and contextual issues in supervision.

The geographic diversity of contributors serves as metaphor for the multitude of supervisory theories and experiences included in this volume. The editors, along with John de Carteret, set a tone of exploration in the first section entitled, "The Evolution of Supervision" by overviewing supervision in terms of Bateson's stochastic model. Supervision is seen as evolving through a repetitive process of interaction, selection, and consolidation.

The section on special techniques of supervision considers videotape, earphones and the supervision group behind a one-way mirror. The first chapter of this section by Monica McGoldrick creatively combines several directive models of therapy with family-of-origin procedures to form a unique approach to supervision. There are also two chapters with a strong focus on conducting live supervision in the same room with the therapist and family. In light of the fact that so few therapeutic facilities have observation rooms, these chapters are particularly useful. The therapeutic application of the supervisory team is also described.

The learning process section features a chapter on the role of analogical and digital

129

communication, a topic important for training as well as therapy. Unfortunately, this chapter neglects to provide an example in a training context. Two chapters examine the learning process from the viewpoint of the trainees, a refreshing perspective treated developmentally from beginning therapist to experienced therapist to trainer. An integration of theory is attempted by Helm Stierlin, Michael Wirsching and Gunthard Weber from the Division of Psychoanalysis and Family Therapy from the University of Heidelberg. From a country where the ideas of Freud are held in high regard, five central concepts emerge that shape both therapy and training. The resulting interventions take the form of either "encounters" (insight) or "strategic work" (a la Milan). The last chapter in this section is the most intriguing contribution of the book. Gill Gorell Barnes and David Campbell, two accomplished therapists, supervise one another in their individual specialties: structural and strategic therapies. In addition to an excellent delineation of the two approaches, Barnes and Campbell describe in detail the experience and conceptual bases for giving and receiving supervision within each model.

The fourth section of the book associates supervisory methods with specific conceptual frameworks. Italy is well represented by the Milan model of supervision with its extensive discussions of family process and positive connotation. Maurizio Andolfi's provocative supervision from the Family Therapy Institute of Rome seems particularly effective in preventing therapists from becoming enmeshed in rigid family systems. From the United Kingdom, Brian Cade and Philippa Seligman of the Family Institute from Wales label their conceptual framework "strategic" but describe basic principles involving the "rules" and interactions of the family system. In some quarters such principles would be considered more structural than strategic. (The editors warned of possible definitional discrepancies in their introduction, stating their policy is to let each chapter establish its own set of labels.) The last conceptual framework, by Chris Hatcher of San Francisco, employs a Double Axis Model. One axis represents the family over time from past to future. The other axis concerns the orientation of the family from task to personal activities. In six stages, the family's progress is charted over the four arms of these two axes.

The last section addresses contextual issues in supervision. Karl Tomm and Lorraine Wright of Calgary train family therapists in a university medical center supported by the Canadian government. The facilities are enviable and the content of their training includes circular pattern diagramming. Levels of competence determine a clear and useful hierarchy within the training program. In another article, Elsa Broder and Leon Sloman of Toronto compare the training of three different groups: psychiatric residents, probation officers and mental health professionals. The learning styles of each are considered. Another training program has been designed around a family day care unit at Marlborough Hospital, England, by Alan Cooklin and David Reeves, who pose advantages and problems unique to that setting.

Those who are doing family therapy supervision will find this book valuable because it stimulates thoughts beyond the usual scope of articles or books on supervision. As the antithesis of a handbook, this volume challenges supervisors to think through the limits they have ascribed to their own facilities and encourages them to consider new possibilities.

MARK J. HIRSCHMANN, M.S., R.N.
Doctoral Student
Marriage and Family Therapy Program
Purdue University
West Lafayette, IN 47907

FROM THE INSIDE OUT AND OTHER METAPHORS: CREATIVE AND IN-
TEGRATIVE APPROACHES TO TRAINING IN SYSTEMS THINKING. Duhl, B.
(1983), *New York: Brunner/Mazel, 298 pages.*

The title of this book is intriguing. It provokes the kind of search for meaning associated with the anecdotes of the late Milton Erickson. One is free to conjure up any number
of interesting topics the title could fit. This is dangerous, however, since reality generally
is disappointing when compared to fantasy.

Bunny Duhl reduces this danger by beginning her book with a description of what it is
not. For example, the book is not about doing therapy, nor is it filled with facts and answers. A more descriptive title might be *Training at the Boston Family Institute as Experienced by Bunny Duhl.*

Training at the Boston Family Institute (BFI) is based on the assumption that the "processes in, between, and among trainees" are "analogous to those that occur in families."
The book describes the germination of that assumption and the experiential training procedures developed at BFI.

The volume is divided into three main sections. The first deals with the development of
BFI. This historical perspective traces the emergence of systemic thinking in general and
provides autobiographical sketches of several key BFI trainers, including the author. The
second section discusses the multicentric human systems thinking used at BFI and the
author's assumptions underlying adult human learning. The third section contains provocative discussions of BFI's brand of experiential training.

BFI attempts to create a learning environment sensitive to individual learning styles
where the trainees can experience their self-in-context and derive formulas and a therapeutic style that best fits their unique talents. Thus, learning and observation from the inside (self) can be generalized to the outside (family) systems. BFI trains from the inside
out by offering a variety of experiential exercises designed to break old rules of behavior
and expand options.

A wealth of metaphoric material and guidelines for creating analogic experiences are
contained in this work. For example, the author discusses a variety of family sculpture
procedures applicable to both training and therapy.

In sum, this book is an extremely useful source of creative ideas for anyone interested
in experiential/metaphoric methods of teaching human systems thinking.

ROGER LAIRD, Ed.D.
Barren River Comprehensive Care
707 East Main Street
Bowling Green, KY 42101

Reviews of Training Videotapes

HEROIN MY BABY, produced under the auspices of The Addicts and Families Project of the Philadelphia Child Guidance Clinic and the Philadelphia Veterans Administration Hospital Drug Dependence Treatment Center, M. Duncan Stanton, Project Director, Thoman C. Todd, Project Consultant. *Videotape, 3/4" b&w cassette, 40 minutes. Purchase or rental from Family Therapy Institute, 5850 Hubbard Dr., Rockville, Md. 20852. One week rental, $100; purchase, $325.*

This videotape demonstrates a method of treating heroin addiction using a structural-strategic family therapy approach. Instead of viewing the problem from an individual perspective (e.g., the identified patient has an addictive personality) or from a dyadic perspective (e.g., the individual takes drugs to stay involved with his mother), this approach conceptualizes the problem from a triadic perspective. The underlying premise of this approach posits that parents communicate through their troubled child and stay together because of him/her. When the son in this videotape begins to succeed and leave home, the parents face only each other and threaten to seperate. Then the son fails (i.e., takes drugs) and pulls the parents back together to take care of him. The goal of therapy is twofold: first, move the son out of the marriage, and second, establish an appropriate hierarchy whereby the parents deal with an irresponsible son.

This conceptualization of the problem and the concomitant therapeutic interventions are clearly and graphically illustrated. Attainment of the first goal of therapy, moving the addicted son out of the marriage, is illustrated by two therapeutic moves. In the first, the therapist physically moves the son out from between the parents and places himself between the couple. This not only begins the process of extricating the son from the marital relationship, but it also communicates to the family that the therapist is in charge, a message which must be accepted if goal two is to be achieved and therapy is to be successful. The second intervention entails having the parents communicate with each other about their son without allowing the son to intrude. As the parents begin to talk, their recurring, homeostatic family pattern is illustrated. The couple begin to talk, their discussion develops into an argument, and the son interrupts their arguing and redirects their attention to him. Consequently, the parents avoid ever dealing with their conflicts. This sequence and the therapist's moves to block the son's intrusion are clearly illustrated. The second goal, establishing a correct hierarchy, is the major therapeutic intervention of therapy. As in the case of the first goal, this goal is achieved through a series of well defined and clearly illustrated therapeutic moves. The moves include: (a) establishing a contract between therapist and couple which states that the parents agree to work together on the problem, (b) creating the reality that the parents represent joint authorities over the son, (c) asking the more peripheral parent to take charge of the son while having the more involved parent communicate to his/her spouse rather than to the son, and (d) persuading and coaching the parents to give their son up. As the parental subsystem becomes more cohesive and functional, the therapist gradually moves himself out of the system, allowing it to establish its own new patterns.

This tape is a studio-produced enactment based exclusively on transcripts of an actual family in therapy. Family members are portrayed by skilled professional actors. The therapist on the tape is the same therapist who worked on the original case. The simulations are well-acted, effectively photographed, and tightly edited. Moreover, the narration, performed by Jay Haley, is clear and well-timed.

The use of the videotape for training purposes has merit. The tape illustrates Haley's

Problem Solving approach to therapy in an effective, interesting manner. Consequently, this videotape would be a useful addition to a course curriculum on structural/strategic therapy.

NICHOLAS S. ARADI, Ed.S.
Doctoral Student
Marriage and Family Therapy Program
Purdue University
West Lafayette, IN 47907

THE DAUGHTER WHO SAID NO, videotape, 3/4" b&w cassette, 70 minutes (two parts). *Rental from The Ackerman Institute for Family Therapy, 149 East 78 St., New York, N.Y. 10021. One week rental $140.*

This videotape illustrates the practice of systemic therapy, Ackerman Institute-style. A fundamental assumption of this approach states that change occurs by establishing a particular structure in therapy. The structure consists of a therapeutic triangle represented by the therapist, the family, and the consultation group. The consultation group is comprised of the therapist's colleagues who observe the therapy from behind a one way mirror. It is this therapeutic triangle around which negotiations for change take place. The major interventions utilized during negotiations are paradoxical interventions and input from the consultation group.

The case chosen to demonstrate this approach is a family in which a child has anorexia nervosa. The family consists of parents in their early fifties and three daughters in their twenties. The youngest daughter, age 23, is anorexic, and was referred by an internist for family therapy. Peggy Papp is the therapist and Olga Silverstein is the consultant on the case. The tape is not an enactment, but a compilation of the actual therapy sessions spanning a one year period.

Unlike many videotape presentations of systemic therapy which tend to be rich in drama and intrigue, but weak in specificity and explanation, this presentation is rich in both.

The case example used to illustrate the approach is fascinating. The presenting problem is chronic and life threatening, the family depicted is expressive and spirited, and the therapeutic interventions are brilliantly conceived and artistically implemented. All of this combine to make viewing enjoyable and fascinating. However, the quality which sets this presentation apart from others on systemic therapy is its systematic and comprehensive explanation of the therapy process.

The tape is divided in two parts, each part being further organized into stages of therapy. Each stage is first identified using graphics, then illustrated by showing scenes of the therapy session, and finally processed by a brief narration which presents the rationale for each intervention. Stages in Part One include "Forming a Hypothesis", "Connecting the Symptom with the System", "Dealing with Change", "Fall-Out from Change", and "Enlisting the Sibling Subsystem". Part Two continues with "Saying No to Therapy", "Solidifying Change", and "Celebrating Independence".

While not explicitly stated, Part One of the tape illustrates first order change and Part Two shows second order change. At the end of part one, the presenting problem is solved as the daughter begins to eat and gain weight. However, family relationships are unaltered. The system remains unchanged. Part Two documents second order change. The daughter is moved to rebel against the parent-child relationship she's maintained with her parents, and struggles to establish her independence. In the process, the parents renegotiate their relationship as they learn to live their lives without her. As these relationships change, the family system evolves to a quantitatively different level of organization.

This is an informative, interesting tape which possesses several strengths for use in training. Most importantly, it clearly identifies key concepts and techniques of systemic therapy. In addition, it illustrates the way in which a specific family problem is conceptualized in terms of key principles. Lastly, the tape shows the implementation of techniques and interventions unique to systemic therapy. One limitation of this tape is the fact that no attention is given to the process by which interventions are developed. A segment showing what goes on behind the one-way mirror—among the consultation group and/or between the therapist and the group—would have been useful. Overall, though, this tape is well worth seeing.

NICHOLAS S. ARADI, Ed.S.
Family Therapy Program
Purdue University
West Lafayette, IN 47907

ASSESSMENT AND INTERVENTION STRATEGIES IN FAMILY THERAPY, by Anita Menfi, Director of the Family Psychiatric Center, Albert Einstein College of Medicine, New York. *Videotape, 3/4" color cassette, 60 minutes. Purchase or rental from IEA Production, Inc., 520 East 77th Street, New York, NY 10021. Three day rental $125; purchase $235. (All other video formats available on request.)*

The title of this videotape is misleading. It suggests that the viewer will be presented an overview of existing assessment procedures and intervention strategies in the field of family therapy. In fact, what is presented is an explication of a particular type of family therapy. A more appropriate title for this videotape is "An Introduction to Family Crisis Therapy".

The tape is loosely organized into four sections. In section one, the purpose and goals of Family Crisis Therapy (FCT) are defined, its format is described, and four questions which structure and guide the therapy are identified. Section two consists of a 25-minute simulation demonstrating FCT. The simulation is based on a transcript of an initial therapy session with an actual family in crisis. In section three, key principles and concepts of Family Crisis Therapy are identified and illustrated by repeating segments of the therapy session. In the last section, the four questions integral to Family Crisis Therapy are reviewed and answered in terms of the family depicted.

Anita Menfi, Direrctor of the Family Studies Section of the Bronx Psychiatric Center, and presumable originator of FCT, is both therapist and narrator on the tape. She begins the presentation by describing FCT as a short-term (six week) intervention designed to treat families which seek to hospitalize a schizophrenic family member. The goal of FCT is to avert hospitalization and involve the family in brief, intensive family therapy. The therapy attempts to restructure the family's life so that it can mobilize its own coping skills to meet the crisis situation. It is implied that FCT was developed and is most appropriately implemented in a hospital setting. Monfi ends her overview of FCT by asking the viewer to consider the following four key questions while watching the simulated case presentation:

1. What are the functional characteristics of the family?
2. What specific information is necessary?
3. What is the primary crisis in the family?
4. What therapeutic interventions would you make?

Section two, the simulation of a first session in Family Crisis Therapy, begins with an abbreviated genogram to introduce the family. This white, anglo, middle class family is comprised of a husband and wife in their late 40's and their three children, two daughter, ages 21 and 20, and a son, age 19. The family sought to hospitalize the son for acting "bizarre"; but, instead, were referred by the hospital for family therapy.

Essentially, the enactment portrays a family in crisis over separation. The simulation reveals a disengaged and conflictual marital relationship, a highly enmeshed mother/daughter relationship, and a family myth which dictates that women are successful and competent, and men are losers. As the younger daughter attempts to disengage from her mother by moving into her own apartment, the son prevents the move by acting out and, thereby, creating a crisis which stabilizes the family system.

In section three, key principles and guidelines of Family Crisis Therapy are examined. The method utilized to do this is interesting and effective. The principle is first stated, then demonstrated by showing the appropriate segment of the therapy session just viewed. While numerous practical structuring, relationship, and theoretical principles are explicated, they are done so in a seemingly unsystematic and arbitrary manner. They are presented in terms of their sequence on the tape, rather than on the basis of any underlying theory. Moreover, the principles presented represent a virtual potpourri of concepts from a variety of family therapies. Some of the theories from which the principles are drawn include Structural (importance of identifying subsystems), strategic (emphasis on information gathering and creating a "problem-solving frame"), functional (importance of the therapist assuming a managerial role), and Hill's ABCX stress model (emphasis of family stressors and activating the family's coping mechanisms). While the principles appear to be effective, they are presented without rationale. Consequently, the viewer is exposed to a plethora of principles without any sort of schema or theoretical framework by which to organize and integrate them.

In the last section, the four key questions of FCT are reviewed and answered. The method used to present this information is the same as that used in the introduction section—a close-up image of the narrator talking to the viewer. Both sections contained interesting information presented in an uninteresting way. The use of graphics during these sections would have helped maintain the viewer's interest and facilitated his/her learning.

From an instructional standpoint, this videotape has several limitations. Most problematic is the absence of a clear statement of objectives. This leaves the viewer without any clear sense as to the direction of the presentation. Moreover, the absence of a clearly articulated theoretical framework, no mention of FCT's application to nonhospital settings, and the failure to define who/what makes up the "therapy team" (a term used throughout the videotape), contribute greatly to the presentation's ambiguity.

On the positive side, the tape clearly illustrates effective interviewing and structuring techniques. In addition, the tape demonstrates a concrete, problem-focused approach to averting hospitalization of an identified patient in a family experiencing crisis.

NICHOLAS S. ARADI, Ed.S.
Family Therapy Program
Purdue University
West Lafayette, IN 47907

A FAMILY INTERVIEW: A TRAINING PACKAGE IN FAMILY THERAPY WITH VIDEOTAPE, by Douglas C. Breunlin, Institute for Juvenile Research, Celia J. Falicov, University of California, Agnes D. Lattimer, Chicago Medical School and Cook County Hospital, Vajendra J. Desai, University of Illinois and Cook County Hospital. *Videotape available in any format, 35 minutes. Purchase or rental from Center for Educational Development, University of Illinois at the Medical Center, Chicago, Illinois. Three day rental=$75; Purchase=$300.*

A FAMILY THERAPY ASSESSMENT EXERCISE. Instrument by Douglas Breunlin and Richard Schwartz, both of the Institute for Juvenile Research; based on the above videotape by Breunlin et al. *Videotape available in any format, 60 minutes. Purchase or rental from Center for Educational Development, University of Illinois at the Medical Center, Chicago, Illinois. Three day rental=$75; Purchase =$300.*

Both of the above videotapes are of the same therapy session, one being continous (A Family Interview: A Training Package in Family Therapy), the other broken up into brief segments (A Family Therapy Assessment Exercise) to allow time for respondents to answer questions on a multiple-choice instrument to measure therapists' competency in structural therapy. The 35 minute interview was developed from an actual initial family therapy session conducted by Celia Falicov. Actors were hired to re-enact the script. Realism is high, providing the viewer with the type of stimulus that a therapist would typically encounter. A wide range of interventions are illustrated and family dynamics of moderate complexity are depicted. Some modifications from the actual therapy session were incorporated to highlight important conceptual material and to include therapist behaviors which could be thought of as clinical errors.

The authors suggest that the training package, which consists of the videotape and an accompanying training manual, be used by beginning and intermediate level students who have an interest in family therapy. The training package can be used either with or without a supervisor/trainer. The suggested progression of the training involves, first, an introduction to a structural conceptual framework, enabling the viewer to understand the functioning of family systems and appropriate intervention strategies. (This information is presented in the manual, not the videotape.) Following the reading of this introductory material, the videotape is to be viewed and discussed in relation to the structural conceptual material presented. Next, a narrated transcript of the family therapy interview with observational comments (also included in the manual) is intended to be used to provide a more detailed analysis of both family dynamics and therapeutic interventions. Finally, the authors suggest that the videotape be viewed again to maximize one's learning.

As a training tool, the package is quite useful. The fact that the authors have chosen a singular model and have provided a systematic and practical presentation of the conceptual information is to be commended. The result is an effective interplay between the conceptual underpinnings and the practical execution of structural therapy.

The authors' inclusion of therapeutic "mistakes" also makes for an interesting twist. Because these have been included, there is the potential for greater discussion and evaluation from viewers without the intimidation that all therapeutic interventions are presumed to be "best" or "right" (as one might presume by watching the edited videotapes of wizards like Minuchin, Papp, or Haley). Moreover, rationales and criticisms of therapist behavior are enumerated in the written transcript and subsequent discussion.

One drawback of the videotape is that the actors often do not precisely generate the timing, spontaneity, and emotions of a real family in pain. While not nullifying the tape's value, it does mildly detract from its overall quality.

The second videotape, which is the same session but in the discontinuous format, is presently being developed to accompany a written assessment instrument. The instrument, used in conjunction with showing the videotaped segments, has been designed to assess three inter-related sets of skills: observational, conceptual and therapeutic. These are virtually the same as Cleghorn and Levin's (1973) perceptual, conceptual and executive skills. Observational skills are those required to perceive and accurately describe behavioral data within a session. Conceptual skills reflect a theoretical understanding of a model. Therapeutic skills are those necessary to execute interventions skillfully within the session according to one's model of therapy, in this case structural. The instrument (Breunlin et al., 1983) is intended to provide a measure of a trainee's competence in these three sets of skills.

The instrument has been constructed with jargon-free language, which allows those unfamiliar with family therapy terminology to understand each item and insures that the test measures more than the respondents' acquaintance with the vocabulary of the structural model. But, due to its reliance upon the structural model, Breulin et al. (1981, 1983) acknowledge that it is theoretically possible that a highly trained clinician from a contrasting school might do very poorly on this test.

With a multiple-choice format, the test is easy to score. Moreover, preliminary studies suggest that the instrument dos not suffer from either "basement" or "ceiling" effects (respondents skewing toward the low or high end of the scale). Earlier versions of the instrument have exhibited discriminant validity (see Breunlin et al., 1983), but further reliability and validity studies are needed.

In addition to the instrument's capacity to assess therapists' skills, it may be used as an excellent training tool. For example, a trainee can systematically build his/her knowledge by taking the test, then reading the manual, and possibly observing the videotape again. Another option is, of course, to use the assessment instrument as a pre- and post-test to assess acquired competency in structural family therapy gained by other training packages/formats. The uses are multiple and they range from formal assessment to informal, self-structured training.

REFERENCES

Breunlin, D., Lattimer, A., Desai, V. & Falicov, C. (1981). A family interview: A training manual in family therapy, Center for Educational Development, University of Illinois at the Medical Center.

Breunlin, D. C., Schwartz, R. C., Krause, M. S., Selby, L. M. (1983). Evaluating family therapy training: The development of an instrument. *Journal of Marital and Family Therapy, 9,* 37-48.

Cleghorn, J. & Levin, S. (1973). Training family therapists by setting learning objectives. *American Journal of Orthopsychiatry, 43,* 439-446.

KAREN HERNANDEZ, M.S.
Family Therapy Program
Purdue University
West Lafayette, IN 47907

Annotated Bibliography
of Key Articles on the Supervision
and Training of Family Therapists*

Marcia Sandridge Brown
Mark J. Hirschmann
John H. Lasley
Cricket K. Steinweg

I. OVERVIEWS

Liddle, H.A. (1982). Family therapy training: Current issues, future trends. *International Journal of Family Therapy, 4,* 31-97.

This article extrapolates five realms of focus from previous literature on family therapy training: a) personnel, b) content, c) methodology, d) context, and e) evaluation. Corresponding to each domain the following questions are raised: 1) Who should teach or be taught family therapy? 2) What should be taught? 3) How should the content be taught? 4) How do the training system and training methods influence each other?, and 5) How should training be assessed? The article thoroughly examines controversial issues in training which have yet to be resolved. While the author shows some bias for learning from a particular theory versus eclecticism, he otherwise attempts to present both sides of the issues.

Liddle, H.A. (1982). On the problems of eclecticism: A call for epistemologic clarification and human-scale theories. *Family Process, 21,* 243-250.

This paper examines several theoretical issues facing family therapists: a) competitive struggles among schools of therapy for followers, b) limits to what one can know with any theory, c) problems with eclecticism, including its role and scope, and d) a proposed method for aiding therapists in the process of clarifying and refining their basic beliefs. The author challenges clinicians to avoid loose usage of the word "eclectic" and spurs them on the elucidate issues related to their theory and practice.

Liddle, H.A. & Halpin, R.J. (1978). Family therapy training and supervision literature: A comparative review. *Journal of Marriage and Family Counseling, 4,* 77-98.

This overview compares and categorizes the prevailing family therapy training and supervision literature by focusing upon six areas: a) goals of training/supervision and su-

---

Marcia Sandridge Brown, M.S.W., Mark J. Hirschmann, R.N., John H. Lasley, M.S., and Cricket K. Steinweg, R.N., are doctoral students in the Family Therapy Program, Department of Child Development and Family Studies, Purdue University, West Lafayette, IN 47907.

*Appears in a different form in Piercy, F. and Sprenkle, D. (in press). *Family therapy sourcebook.* New York: Guilford.

pervisor skills, b) supervisory techniques, c) the supervisor-supervisee relationship, d) personal therapy for trainees, e) politics of family therapy training, and f) evaluation. Gaps in the literature, both conceptual and empirical, are identified. Over 100 references are categorized within a comprehensive table, making this article a handy resource.

Okun, B. & Gladding, S. (Eds.), (1983). *Issues in training marriage and family therapists.* Ann Arbor, MI: ERIC/CAPS.

This monograph of the Association of Counselor Education and Supervision (ACES) focuses on relevant family therapy training issues relevant to counselor educators. There are several good articles on training and supervision. One article suggests a creative alternative to the either-or issue of family therapy as a profession or a professional speciality, and another identifies some important gender issues relevant to training family therapists.

Simon, R. & Brewster, F. (1983). What is training? *Family Therapy Networker, 7*(2), 25-29, 66.

The authors of this article take a human-interest approach to the topic of training. They identify five phases a student in any training program might encounter, emphasizing the feelings that such a process may arouse. This article is peppered with interesting quotes from leaders in the field that reveal their dilemmas with family therapy and supervision. The article is not intended to be a rigorous discourse on training but rather an evocative experience with the subject matter, putting the reader in touch with the emotional issues involved from either side of the one-way mirror.

II. LIVE SUPERVISION

Berger, M. & Dammann, C. (1982). Live supervision as context, treatment, and training. *Family Process, 21,* 337-344.

The uniqueness of this contribution lies in the willingness of the authors to examine not only the advantages of live supervision but also the potential pitfalls. The article addresses the inevitable struggle between the perceptions of therapist and supervisor which originate from opposite sides of the one-way screen. In addition, the value of varying perspectives is lauded and the synthesis of multi-views is recommended for enhanced treatment and training.

Beroza, R. (1983). The shoemaker's children. *Family Therapy Networker, 7*(2), 31-33.

This essay takes the stand that live supervision has sufficiently come of age to no longer be just the political symbol for directive versus traditional therapy, but also to be justly deserving of constructive criticism. The main caution offered is that a therapist may not always emerge confident from a session with live supervision. The author's tack is likely to be highly useful to supervisors struggling to define their roles with therapists-in-training.

Coopersmith, E.I. (1980). Expanding uses of the telephone in family therapy. *Family Process, 19,* 411-417.

Creative uses of the telephone in family therapy are described. The author gives examples of calls to the therapist, calls from the team to specific family members, and calls between family members. These case examples demonstrate the impact of the format on recalcitrant families. The author additionally shows how she simultaneously capitalizes on use of the team for both therapeutic and training purposes.

Papp, P. (1980). The Greek chorus and other techniques of paradoxical therapy. *Family Process, 19,* 45-57.

This important article describes the process of paradoxical family therapy, including the indications, principles, and limitations of such techniques as reframing, prescription, and reversals. The "Greek Chorus" (the supervisory team) is highlighted as useful to several paradoxical interventions appropriate for a family resistant to change. This article is rich in examples and is a prime source for family therapists interested in live supervision and/or paradoxical intervention strategies.

III. SUPERVISORY SKILLS/TECHNIQUES

Constantine, J.A., Stone Fish, L. & Piercy, F.P. (1984). A systematic procedure for teaching positive connotation. *Journal of Marital and Family Therapy, 10*(3), 313-316.

A unique step-by-step approach is proposed for teaching trainees the strategic technique of circumventing family resistance via positive connotation of noxious behavior. The training procedure is group-oriented and systematically moves from brainstorming, to contributions behind a one-way mirror, to generalization in therapy. The brief nature of the article makes for easy introductory reading.

Garrigan, J.J. & Bambrick, A.F. (1977). Introducing novice therapists to "go-between" techniques of family therapy. *Family Process, 16*(2), 237-246.

This paper identifies the competencies, objectives, and evaluation criteria used in a program to train therapists in Zuk's "go-between" method of family therapy. This was one of the first family training programs to carefully identify operationalizable objectives. The authors' method of graphically articulating competencies with corresponding perceptual/conceptual and therapeutic skills, as well as criteria for evaluating these skills, is a useful paradigm for family therapy trainers to consider.

Heath, A.W. & Storm, C.L. (1983). Answering the call: A manual for beginning supervisors. *Family Therapy Networker, 7*(2), 36-37, 66.

This highly readable article contains a set of guidelines for the family therapist who is assuming supervisory responsibility for the first time. The authors urge the development of a conceptual framework of supervision based, in part, on the similarities of therapy and supervision. This "manual" to supervision also offers a supplemental list of readings to compensate for its brevity.

Liddle, H.A. (1982). Using mental imagery to create therapeutic and supervisory realities. *The American Journal of Family Therapy, 10,* 68-72.

This is a short but potent article which reminds supervisors to create experiential bridges for their supervisees through the use of visual and auditory imagery. The thoughts presented are innovative and provocative and set the mind spinning in new directions. This is an unusually analogic style for the author and the content will likely be a refreshing addition to a supervisor's repertoire.

Liddle, H.A. & Schwartz, R.C. (1983). Live supervision/consultation: Conceptual and pragmatic guidelines for family therapy trainers. *Family Process, 22,* 477-490.

In this article the authors provide a rather thorough list of live supervision skills. These skills could be useful to supervisors in developing live-supervision learning objectives and/or evaluation tools.

Roberts, J. (1983). The third tier: The overlooked dimension in family therapy training. *The Family Therapy Networker, 7*(2), 30-31, 60-61.

A case is presented for the field of family therapy to now "appreciate the importance of the larger therapeutic-educational system that includes the supervisor, therapist, family, and the group of trainees behind the one-way mirror." The author identifies supervisory responsibilities in developing a "collaborative team" which will expand the potential of the training group. Some of the training techniques suggested are likely to be controversial in that team trainees may be left unsupervised to rise to the occasion on their own.

IV. FAMILY THERAPY EDUCATION AND TRAINING

Cade, B.W. & Seligman, P.M. (1982). Teaching a strategic approach. In R. Whiffen and J. Byng-Hall (Eds.), *Family therapy supervision: Recent developments in practice* (pp. 167-179). New York: Grune & Stratton.

General interactional and systemic principles underlie strategic therapy and live supervision. Family and trainee behavioral change are enhanced through the extension of interactional skills, especially through the use of humor. A set of examples demonstrates the versatility of this style of supervision and provides introductory ideas to the novice family therapy trainer.

Liddle, H.A. & Saba, G.W. (1982). Teaching family therapy at the introductory level: A conceptual model emphasizing a pattern which connects training and therapy. *Journal of Marital and Family Therapy, 8,* 63-72.

An introductory family therapy course evolving over six years is thoroughly outlined. The parallel nature of the processes of teaching and therapy are emphasized. Three stages of this course—joining, restructuring, and consolidation—focus upon the issue of working from a systemic point of view with trainees. Fundamental issues for trainers in family therapy are raised for consideration and a suggested final examination is included for those planning similar courses.

Piercy, F.P. & Sprenkle, D.H. (1983). Ethical, legal, and professional issues in family therapy: A graduate level course. *Journal of Marital and Family Therapy, 9*(4), 393-401.

This presentation of a sixteen-week academic course in ethical, legal, and professional issues facing family therapists may be used as a model for training clinicans in real-life dilemmas typically not described in texts. In addition, students are offered assignments and experiential activities geared to promote their own professional development. While the authors concede that the topics covered are not comprehensive, the course is global enough in focus that the sources introduced provide a solid foundation and launching pad for exploring related considerations.

Piercy, F.P. & Sprenkle, D.H. (Equal Authorship) (1984). The process of family therapy education. *Journal of Marital and Family Therapy, 10*(4), 399-407.

Suggestions for the process of graduate family therapy education are prefaced with theoretical assumptions promoting student involvement and critical evaluation of seminal works in the field. Examples of course assignments intended to synergize theory, research, and practice are included along with multiple assessment methods for capitalizing upon student strengths. This is a prime source for family therapy trainers seeking to expand their existing modes of instruction.

Prosky, P. (1983). The use of analogic and digital communication in training systems perception and intervention. In R. Whiffen and J. Byng-Hall (Eds.), *Family therapy supervision: Recent developments in practice,* (109-113). New York: Grune & Stratton.

Prosky suggests that incongruencies of analogical and digital communication serve as indicators of systemic dysfunction. Trainers are encouraged to help trainees to maintain consistency between verbal and nonverbal behaviors and to extend their analogical range by using metaphoric messages and sculpting techniques. The chapter's most important contribution is the call to investigate the interface between the communicative behaviors of therapist and family in treatment.

Sprenkle, D.H. & Piercy, F.P. (1984). Research in family therapy: A graduate level course. *Journal of Marital and Family Therapy, 10*(3), 225-240.

This guide to developing a thorough graduate course in family therapy research is rich in examples from a teaching repertoire designed to ease student anxiety about the subject, provide exposure to existing studies/assessment tools, and foster interest in the prevailing issues. Traditional methods of teaching are juxtaposed with more discovery-oriented modalities. Of particular significance is a section developed to acquaint budding researchers with the dilemmas of how to measure systemic change as opposed to change in individual family members.

Tomm, K. & Wright, L. (1982). Multilevel training and supervision in an outpatient service program. In R. Whiffen and J. Byng-Hall (Eds.), *Family therapy supervision: Recent developments in practice,* (pp. 211-227). New York: Grune & Stratton.

This chapter articulates many of the policies and procedures adopted at the family therapy program at the University of Calgary. Training facilities, content of training, levels of training, methods of training, and evaluation methods are covered. The hallmark of this piece is the authors' discussion of circular pattern diagramming as a teaching tool.

Winkle, C.W., Piercy, F.P. & Hovestadt, A.J. (1981). A curriculum for graduate-level marriage and family therapy education. *Journal of Marital and Family Therapy.* 7(2), 201-210.

This study, employing the Delphi technique to approach consensus among AAMFT Approved Supervisors and training directors, compares subjects' choices of topics to be covered in a graduate-level family therapy training program with those recommended by AAMFT guidelines. Areas of overlap and points of disagreement are noted with the expressed purpose of providing feedback to educators and practitioners in the field. This is a quality source for those planning or re-evaluating training programs and for those wanting to identify areas for independent study to fill in gaps in their own educational background.

V. SUPERVISION OF SUPERVISION

Constantine, J.A., Piercy, F.P. & Sprenkle, D.H. (1984). Supervision of supervision. *Journal of Marital and Family Therapy, 10,* 95-97.

This brief report concentrates on the live supervision of the supervisor-in-training. A multi-tiered supervisory process is described and the issues "as one moves up the hierarchy" are delineated. Of special interest is the authors' analysis of their past mistakes which interfered with clear differentiation of roles between therapist, supervisor, and meta-supervisor.

Heath, A.W. & Storm, C.L. (In press). From the institute to the Ivory Tower: The live supervision stage approach for teaching supervision in academic settings. *American Journal of Family Therapy.*

This article describes the components of Purdue's course in family therapy supervision, which combines a supervision seminar and practicum and culminates in students' live supervision of live supervision. This is a good resource for anyone planning such a course.

Liddle, H.A., Breunlin, D.C., Schwartz, R.C. & Constantine, J.A. (1984). Training family therapy supervisors: Issues of content, form, and context. *Journal of Marital and Family Therapy 10*(2), 139-150.

This paper elaborates on the form, structure and process of a program to train family therapy supervisors in the live supervision of structural-strategic therapy. The program includes a small group supervision seminar, individual supervision-of-supervision meetings, and a supervision group which involves the direct observation/supervision of a supervisor-trainee's work. This article would be quite useful for anyone involved in supervision of supervision.

VI. FAMILY THERAPY SKILLS

Cleghorn, J.M. & Levin, S. (1973). Training family therapists by setting learning objectives. *American Journal of Orthopsychiatry, 43,* 439-446.

The authors of this article exhibit considerable clarity in distinguishing behavioral objectives for basic level, advanced, and experienced family therapists. Distinctions between the proposed categories of perceptual, conceptual, and executive skills are less clear, although the classification is cited widely in the family therapy training literature. Therapists who are making the transition from individual therapy to systemic modalities will find this source particularly valuable, as will their trainers.

Falicov, C.J., Constantine, J.A. & Breunlin, D.C. (1981). Teaching family therapy: A program based on training objectives. *Journal of Marital and Family Therapy, 7,* 497-505.

This paper represents an initial step in identifying family therapy training objectives toward the goal of training evaluation. Observational, conceptual, and therapeutic skills are delineated for a direct, problem-solving family therapy approach. The authors concede that the curriculum components in their training program probably overlap and should be integrated in practice more than their list of objectives would suggest.

Tomm, K.M. & Wright, L.M. (1979). Training in family therapy: Perceptual, conceptual, and executive skills. *Family Process, 18*(3), 227-250.

A rather thorough link-up between perceptual/conceptual skills and corresponding executive skills is presented with numerous examples for family therapists' use in-session. The model delineates therapist functions, competencies, and skills to be displayed over the course of therapy and provides a handy reference for trainers who wish to underscore the strengths of their trainees as well as areas needing improvement. The bulk of the article is in outline form and may be difficult to absorb in one sitting.

VII. EVALUATION

Barton, C. & Alexander, J.F. (1977). Therapists' skills as determinants of effective systems-behavioral family therapy. *International Journal of Family Counseling, 5,* 11-19.

This article discusses therapy skills which the authors suggest are likely to be related to treatment success. Structuring and relationship skills, in particular, were found to account for 60 percent of the variance in treatment outcome in a previous study. This article provides a useful format for clinicians or supervisors-in-training who are looking for a conceptual framework to evaluate therapist skills rather than just techniques.

Breunlin, D.C., Schwartz, R.C., Krause, M.S. & Selby, L.M. (1983). Evaluating family therapy training: The development of an instrument. *Journal of Marital and Family Therapy, 9,* 37-47.

An instrument for assessing trainees' degree of systemic thinking evolved out of a series of studies to establish content and predictive validity. Family therapy trainees are given questions to answer in response to a studio-produced videotape based upon an actual initial family therapy session. The authors openly discuss the challenges of creating an effective questionnaire which distinguishes skill levels between beginning (linear-thinking) therapists and advanced (circular-thinking) practitioners of family therapy.

Kniskern, D.P. & Gurman, A.S. (1979). Research on training in marriage and family therapy: Status, issues, and directions. *Journals of Marital and Family Therapy, 5,* 83-92.

This overview of the evaluative literature for family therapy training raises many important research questions. The article exposes the "empirical ignorance" associated with gaps in the profession's knowledge base regarding training and is thorough in raising issues for clinicians, supervisors, and researchers alike. The authors pinpoint a variety of uncharted areas ripe for investigation.

Piercy, F.P., Laird, R.A. & Mohammed, Z. (1983). A family therapist rating scale. *Journal of Marital and Family Therapy, 9,* 49-59.

The development and validation of a scale for evaluating family therapist skills is presented. The scale includes five skill categories: Structuring, Relationship, Historical, Structural/Process, and Experiential, each with ten items. An initial validation study found that the scale significantly discriminated between experienced and inexperienced family therapists. Additional psychometric data are presented and possible uses of the scale are discussed.